SalonOvations

Beautiful Black Styles

LOUISE COTTER

SalonOvations

(A Division of Milady Publishing Company)
3 Columbia Circle, Box 12519
Albany, New York 12212–2519

NOTICE TO THE READER

Cover Design: Brian Yacur

Milady Staff
Publisher: Catherine Frangie
Project Editor: Annette Danaher
Production Manager: Brian Yacur
Developmental Editor: Joe Miranda

COPYRIGHT © 1995
by Milady Publishing Company
a division of Delmar Publishers

Printed in the United States of America

For more information, contact:
Milady Publishing Company
3 Columbia Circle , Box 15015
Albany, New York   12212-5015

1 2 3 4 5 6 7 8 9 10 XXX   01 00 99 98 97 96 95

Library of Congress Cataloging-in-Publication Data

Cotter, Louise
      SalonOvations' Beautiful Black Styles/ Louise Cotter
            p.   cm.
         ISBN: 1-56253-222-7
         1. Hairdressing of Afro-Americans.   I. Title
TT972.C68 1995   94-30000
646.7'242'0899673−dc20   CIP

Photo Credits

Photographer

Sally Russ
Orlando, Florida

Makeup Artist

Frieda Valenzuela
Orlando, Florida

Hair Stylists and Technicians

Style 1
> Candi Ekstrom
> HairBenders
> Altamonte Springs, Florida

Styles 2,
> Jill Hagerty
> Orlando, Florida

Styles 3, 4, 6
> Rachel Kangas
> HairBenders
> Altamonte Springs, Florida

Styles 5, 7, 10
> Sara Ringler
> Sara N'Woody's Beauté Center
> Orlando, Florida

Style 12
> Christine Gross
> HairBenders
> Altamonte Springs, Florida

Styles 8, 9, 11
> Vincent Maxwell
> Salon de Leonardo
> Altamonte Springs, Florida

About The Author

LOUISE COTTER is a respected educator and leader in the cosmetology industry. Her dedication to the art of cosmetology is evidenced in her lifelong work as a salon owner, instructor, educational director, editor of a major industry magazine, and author of many educational texts.

Ms. Cotter's educational background provided the fundamentals necessary for communicating on multiple levels of cosmetology. In addition to a wide range of cosmetology skills, her professional expertise extends to art and journalism.

She is a licensed cosmetologist and cosmetology instructor who participates in industry-sponsored events, seminars, and continuing education programs nationwide. She is an accomplished platform artist and lecturer.

Ms. Cotter is also a member of the National Cosmetology Association (NCA). She received the first NCA Award of Achievement for excellence in cosmetology education.

During her ten-year tenure as editor of *American Salon Magazine* she was instrumental in many progressive changes designed to improve the quality of information and education to its readers, some 160,000 salon industry professionals.

As director of education for a chain of cosmetology schools, she authored much of the supplemental material used in their educational systems.

As style director of the National Cosmetology Association's Education and Creative Committee, OHFC/HairAmerica, she was responsible for initiating the first full-size NCA consumer-oriented magazine featuring NCA trends in hairstyles, fashion, and information promoting professional salon services. After a progression of titles, it is presently a semi-annual publication known as *American Looks*.

Ms. Cotter's contributions to the cosmetology industry and related education are numerous. She participated in the creation of seven NCA Trend Releases, twice served as NCA style director, and was a trainer of the 1976 U.S.A. Ladies Olympic Hairstyling Team. Currently she is owner of ADRIAN CREATIVE IMAGES (ACI), a communication and media service company located in Central Florida. Supported by ACI staff, she is editor and producer of NCA's student membership publication, *FCA TODAY*, in its seventh year of publication.

Education and communication are her media; a love of the industry and a sincere wish to perpetuate excellence in cosmetology is her motivation.

Contents

PART II: HAIRSTYLE TECHNICALS

23

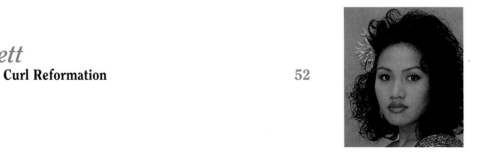

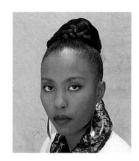
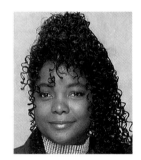
PART III: FINISHED STYLES

Preface

This book is written specifically for cosmetologists seeking information (basic and technically advanced) pertaining to the study of Black hair care.

It is designed to elevate the skills level of cosmetologists, particularly those engaged in professional hair care services to Black women and men, who have a basic knowledge of the subject but wish to become more proficient.

Based on population and economic data, Black, fashion-aware clients spend more discretionary income on personal grooming than any other consumer group. It is also an established fact that sophisticated Black clients will only patronize salons whose staff is knowledgeable and skilled in services vital to their unique hair care needs. Black consumers are not bargain hunters; they are "quality" seekers.

Throughout history, fashion-conscious women have sought to wear currently fashionable hairstyles. The word "fashionable," however, had different interpretations by people of different ethnic backgrounds. Black American women, for instance, wore many traditional hairstyles (not always their preference), even though they didn't have the type of hair necessary to accept and hold most currently changing hairstyles. Their hair needed specific technical care, and technology was slow to respond to those needs.

That is no longer true. Since the early 1950s, high-quality products used to relax and control excessively curly hair, in a safe effective way, has allowed Black women and men to wear hairstyles of their choice. They are no longer limited to styles suitable for their particular hair type. Any hair type can now be easily and safely chemically restructured.

Styling naturally curly hair is a special art that requires knowledge and training beyond basic cosmetology fundamentals. Quoting the accomplished designer, technician, and author, Georgia Calhoun: "Before becoming a master artist, one must master the science which precedes the art."

This BEAUTIFUL BLACK STYLES book addresses all skills necessary to be a designer of Black hairstyles. The most celebrated artists worldwide have never been relegated to just one tool or to any one technique in their effort to create a masterpiece — and neither should you. Progressive cosmetologists must constantly broaden their knowledge, hone their skills, and update the tools used to execute their own masterpieces.

Introduction

The subjects contained in this text are selected because they are the most often used in professional salons that specialize in Black hair care.

The techniques used are modern methods, proven effective by celebrated salon professionals servicing a Black clientele. These professionals give freely of their own styling and technical procedures in order to match your commitment to upgrading your skills, raising your profits, and increasing your career satisfaction.

The styling and chemical and temporary restructuring methods illustrated are directly related to hair texture and desired effect. They will enable you to expand your experience with various tools of the trade and create elegant and practical styles in keeping with current fashion demands.

The first chapters are a quick reference and review of each technique used herein. There is a technical reference number included with each illustrated service. The often quoted adage "the more things change the more they remain the same" bears only a minute ring of truth as related to methods used to control Black hair textures. Giant strides have been made both in styling techniques and the refinement of professional products. Make it part of your continuing education to stay aware and be familiar with the use of new products as they come onto the market.

Part III is composed of finished styles. These full-color photos are for your use – they can be cut from the text and displayed in the salon for your clients. Use this section as a way of promoting all the styles you can create.

While the information contained in this text relates directly to the hair of people of African-American heritage, the same techniques may be used for excessively curly hair of any person regardless of race or color.

Only by continuing to upgrade your basic skills can you hope to reach your highest artistic potential. Once you have executed the styles in this manual you will be able to style the hair of your Black clients with greater confidence.

The technical information in this BEAUTIFUL BLACK STYLES book will hopefully inspire you to be adventurous in creating new hair designs, confident when performing chemical services, and proud in having perfected a craft that offers such satisfaction to you and to the clients you serve.

Part I

TECHNICAL REFERENCE

Shampooing

REFERENCE CODE #101

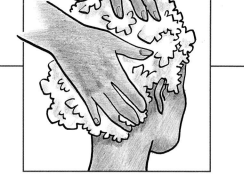

The simple task of cleansing the client's hair and scalp may be the most important service performed in a professional salon; it also may be the most neglected.

It is at the shampoo bowl that the hair is analyzed, cleansed, and conditioned. It is the introductory service on which all your other services will be judged.

In many salons each designer shampoos his own client. This gives you the opportunity to recommend all other services, to educate the client as to the condition of her hair, and an opportunity to sell home maintenance products. All this at the shampoo bowl! The shampoo service is one of the most important services performed in the salon — not because of the money it brings, but because it establishes a good client/salon relationship.

If the shampoo is a pleasant experience for the client — if she feels that every part of her scalp has been massaged, that every strand of hair has been cleansed and rinsed — it will make her a happy, easy-to-deal-with client. If, on the other hand, she feels that she's been given a quick once-over, that the scalp was barely touched, she will be skeptical of all suggested services. And she's well within her right to doubt your expertise in any area, if you don't know how to give a good shampoo.

Aside from selecting the proper type of shampoo, the basic mechanics of a good shampoo should be reviewed from time to time.

For Black clients especially, the scalp should be closely examined for lesions or other disorders. If she is getting a chemical service, perm or relaxer, be certain the manufacturer's instructions allow the hair to be cleansed before the treatment. Most modern products require the application be made on hair free from residue. They do however, warn against unusual stimulation to the scalp.

Just remember, the success of any chemical service depends entirely on three factors:
1. Proper hair analysis
2. Proper product selection
3. Skillful application

Shampoo products are formulated specifically for hair that is dry, oily, damaged, or excessively soiled. Be sure you select a shampoo product based on the hair type and its individual characteristics.

SELECTING THE RIGHT SHAMPOO

Like soaps and detergents, shampoos are cleansing agents. The good ones, however, leave the hair soft, shining, and smooth, particularly if selected for the hair's character — dry, oily, or normal.

Conditioning shampoo is a wise choice for relaxed, dry hair when time is limited. In one quick step, the collagen-protein formula cleans, then lightly coats the strands for smoothness and shine. On fine limp hair it imparts extra body. It's best to alternate such products with deeper cleansing formulas. Conditioning shampoo contains protein ingredients capable of coating the hair, which over time may cause unwanted buildup.

Oily hair presents a special problem requiring a deep cleansing product that retards oil flow at the scalp level.

Hair that has been chemically abused must have a body-building formula. While it doesn't cure the problem, it does conceal it until further treatment can become effective.

Some shampoos contain vitamins A, E, and D, which help restore protein, diminish split ends, and eliminate static build-up.

Shampoos are created for the condition of the hair and scalp. There are as many shampoos as there are hair and scalp conditions. Basically, there are four types of shampoo, used for the following conditions:

- Normal hair and scalp
- Chemically treated hair (tinted, permed, relaxed)
- Dry hair and scalp
- Oily scalp (hair has no oil glands)

Cleansing of the hair and scalp is certainly not one of the more glamorous hair care services, but it is one of the most important — especially to the Black client whose hair needs special attention.

Conditioning
REFERENCE CODE #102

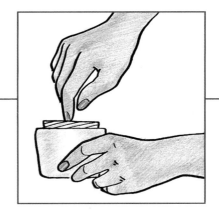

Without going into product detail, it's fair to say few clients have hair that needs no treatment other than shampoo. That would mean the hair has perfect porosity, has no chemical damage, however slight, is free from tangles, has perfect moisture balance, and is sufficiently soft and pliable so the comb glides easily from the scalp to the ends.

Most often the client's hair is too dry, brittle, porous, coated, tangled, broken, or worse. It's up to you to analyze the hair and prescribe the appropriate treatment. Goodness knows there are enough legitimate reasons to recommend a hair/scalp treatment without putting anything on the hair simply to boost the price of the service. Your first priority should always be the well-being of the client.

When you recommend a conditioning treatment of any kind, you should explain to the client the condition of the hair that you believe should be corrected, ingredients the product you recommend contains, and how it will improve the condition of the hair. If a treatment is required, the service should be completed at the time of the shampoo and before the client is directed to the styling station.

Conditioners are formulated with a variety of ingredients and are intended to take over where shampoos leave off. Some conditioners actually remedy problems, while others only offer cosmetic benefits. The therapeutic products help restore and retain moisture, restore lost elasticity, and equalize porosity. The hair then can more easily withstand the tension of combing and brushing and is less likely to be damaged by the application of various chemical processes.

Cosmetic conditioners serve a valid purpose. They enable the hair to look its best at all times, and give instant visible results. Many therapeutic conditioning products offer no immediate results, but instead promise results over a long period of continued use. Dull, damaged hair can benefit temporarily from conditioners that have little but cosmetic value.

Conditioners formulated for severely damaged hair actually penetrate the hair strand, depositing nucleic acids and enzymes that restore the inner structure, improve elasticity, and act to retard excess split and frazzled ends.

Hot oil conditioning formulas seal in natural moisture, which helps prevent the dry brittleness often found in excessively curly hair. Some conditioners contain a combination of vitamins and proteins that gently coat the hair and give a degree of protection while the hair is being groomed. Hot oil conditioners also effectively heighten the shine when used on excessively curly hair.

Some conditioners are formulated to improve the condition of the scalp as well as the hair. They lubricate, eliminating flaking of the scalp and increasing elasticity in the hair.

There are many hair care companies that manufacture products specifically for a Black clientele. The best way to determine which products are the most effective is by using them and comparing the results of each.

For Black clients who want that "wet look" to last all day, use a product especially formulated to be used on a daily basis for this specific purpose.

FACTS ABOUT THE RESULT OF CONDITIONERS ON BLACK HAIR

- Oiling the scalp does not put moisture back into the hair. Oil is a lubricant. It temporarily helps to add shine and pliability, but it does not restore lost moisture to the hair.

- A hair moisturizer, on the other hand, adds and helps retain the moisture already present within the hair. It will also help restore moisture lost due to overexposure to chemicals and/or natural elements.

- It is not true that moisturizers can be applied without first shampooing the hair. It is essential to shampoo first to cleanse the hair and scalp and to open the cuticle of the hair shaft to allow penetration of the moisturizer. Apply moisturizer to extremely wet hair. Black hair has more cuticle layers than that of the average Caucasian. For that reason allow the moisturizer additional time for effective penetration. Adding a heating cap or hot towels will speed up the penetration process. Use a penetrating moisturizer as often as the condition of the hair and scalp dictates. The dryer the hair, the more often it needs to be moisturized.

- It is not true that conditioners eliminate split ends. There are, however, several products made to reduce the appearance of split ends. Actually the frayed or split ends are temporarily fused together, making them less visible. But split ends can only be eliminated by trimming the hair as needed.

HAIR CONDITIONING CAN BE DIVIDED INTO TWO GROUPS — Coating and Penetrating

Coating Conditioners literally coat the hair shaft. They do not penetrate the hair shaft because their molecular structure (size of the molecules) is too large to pass through the openings in the cuticle. This type of conditioner fills the spaces between the cuticle openings and coats the hair shaft, making the hair feel soft and silky. It also helps seal the natural moisture in the hair shaft. Basically this type of conditioner corrects the appearance of the hair but does very little to strengthen its elasticity. Coating conditioners are removed each time the hair is shampooed, therefore, they must be used more often than the penetrating conditioners.

In addition, coating conditioners usually contain a vegetable oil, such as balsam or an animal sub-

stance such as cholesterol. The hair must be rinsed after such conditioner is applied before it is set or styled. Continued used of a coating type conditioner builds up on the hair.

Penetrating Conditioners, just as the name implies, penetrate into the cortex of the hair. The most beneficial of the penetrating conditioners have an acid pH. When a conditioner penetrates into the cortex it helps bond and strengthen damaged cortical fibers. Having an acid pH causes the cuticle to close, helps decrease excess porosity, and adds luster to the hair.

Some penetrating conditioners are left on the hair while others require rinsing before styling. The penetrating qualities of these conditioners usually last through several shampoos.

Penetrating conditioners contain a wide variety of ingredients: animal or vegetable protein, nucleic acids, vitamins, and placenta. It is advisable to follow manufacturer's instructions when using any conditioning product.

HOW TO CORRECTLY APPLY A CONDITIONER

The procedure for applying scalp/hair conditioners varies little. Only the type of conditioner changes. The following is the standard procedure for application. After a thorough cleansing:

- Towel dry the hair and divide into four sections. Place the desired amount of conditioning product on the back of your hand. Make narrow partings and apply product to the scalp with the thumb.
- Manipulate the scalp.
- Cover the hair with a plastic cap, then a heating cap if the treatment calls for it.
- Remove the cap after ten minutes and distribute the conditioner through the hair.
- Reposition the cap and process for as long as necessary to treat the individual condition.
- Remove the cap, rinse thoroughly to remove all product from the hair.

Conditioning treatments, when properly selected and applied, are a valuable salon service. They are beneficial to the client and are an added source of income.

Cutting/Styling

REFERENCE CODE #103

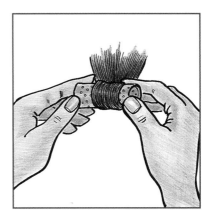

You or some member of your salon staff will have given your client one or more services at the shampoo bowl before she is seated in your styling chair for a haircut and style.

She will have received a shampoo, conditioning treatment, and/or a relaxing service. Any one of those services required you or the technician to make an analysis of the hair type and condition. So when your client is finally seated in your styling chair you are quite familiar with her hair structure.

It is time now to comb through the client's hair. Make a final analysis of the texture, density, and length. Consider the quality and amount of fabric from which you must create a hairstyle.

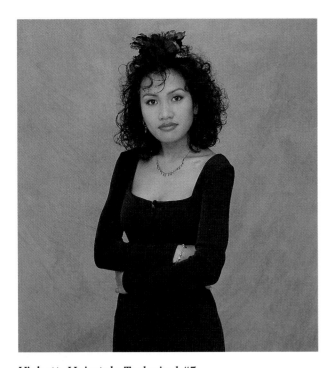

Vichett, Hairstyle Technical #5

Then analyze her facial features. Look at the *profile* for the size and lift of the nose, protrusion or recession of the chin, prominence of the jaw line, and the length and width of the neck. Now look at her "face on" for shape of the face. Is it square, round, rectangular, triangular, or oval? Notice also the span of the forehead, the shape of the eyebrows and whether or not the eyes are close together or wide apart.

Only now can you suggest a hairstyle that is suitable, adaptable, and flattering to your client and one that you know you can deliver based on the amount of hair with which you must work.

Often clients ask for styles that require more hair than they have. For instance, fine, thin hair would not be suitable for luxurious chin-length, blunt bobs or a romantic page boy — even if they are currently fashionable.

Consider also, when recommending a hairstyle to a client, the ease or difficulty she will have maintaining the style between salon appointments. You will be respected much more by your clients if they have an easy time caring for their hair between salon visits.

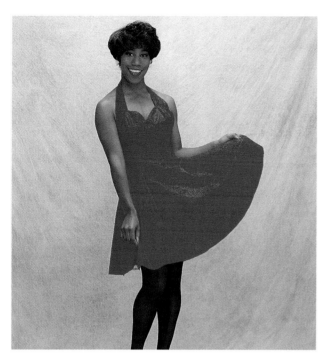

Christine, Hairstyle Technical #8

BLACK HAIR HAS ITS OWN CHARACTERISTICS

Black hair, because of its naturally curly state, has a tendency to be mushy when it is wet and is easily stretched. If too much tension is used when handling, the hair will stretch so it appears longer than it will be when it dries. If you cut to the desired finished length when the hair is wet it is apt to shrink when it dries. That is a terrible disappointment to both you and your client.

For that reason all Black hair should be gently towel blotted until all the excess moisture is removed. Then while it is damp only the stringy ends should be removed, leaving ample length to reshape when the hair is dry. The hair should then be styled by whatever styling method is best for the hair, that is, wet set, blown dry and iron curled, or pressed. When the hair is completely dry brush and comb it to its full length and reshape it during the comb-out.

Often the prudent way to cut Black hair is when it is dry, before the shampoo, especially if the hair is already relaxed or permed to the client's satisfaction. If you do not want to handle hair that is soiled, the hair can first be shampooed, conditioned, blown straight, then cut into the desired style line.

Also, a common practice is to wet set Black hair on very large rollers and put the client under a dryer. When the hair is completely dry, comb and brush it into general lines and cut to desired length. Only then can you be confident the hair will not shrink out of desired form.

BLACK HAIR CAN BE STYLED BY MANY METHODS

- Wet set
- Blow dry and iron curled or set on hot rollers
- Air-formed (blown into style — no ironing)
- Marcel-waves
- Finger-waved, finger-molded, or inch waved
- Braided
- Woven (hair extension)
- (or a combination of any of those methods)

Modern Black women wear very few hair styles simply to make an ethnic statement. Like all women, they are interested in new fashion trends in hair; styles that are adapted to their facial features and body structure; hairstyles that are suitable to their lifestyle, professional and private. Finally, Black women want hairstyles that make them as attractive as they can possibly be.

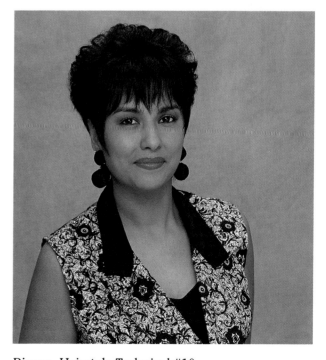

Riaana, Hairstyle Technical #10

Blow Drying/ Air Styling

REFERENCE CODE #104

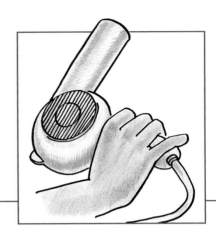

It was once thought the hair of a Black client was unsuitable for "quick service," especially air-styling using a hand-held blow-dryer. With the advent of new technology, products that protect fragile hair are more sophisticated and so are the techniques used to re-form excessively curly hair. It is, indeed, possible to safely and effectively blow-dry Black hair. Often no other tools are needed to complete a beautifully smooth hairstyle.

Blow-drying is the primary technique used for all so-called "quick" services. I downgrade the word "quick," because depending on the condition and length of the hair, styling by blow-drying can be tedious and time consuming.

During the process of blow-drying the physical (hydrogen) bonds are rearranged by using heat and tension on damp hair. When the hair is wet, or damp, it can easily be held with tension with a comb or brush and dried by using a heat source. The heat source must provide a means of completely drying the hair, which makes the hot-air blower an ideal tool. By blowing hot air into narrow panels of curly hair while tension is applied with a comb or brush, the hair is texturally reformed to be straight. Each strand must be thoroughly dry before moving on to additional panels. While tension is important to the drying process, it is important not to overstretch the hair.

The straight effect after blow-drying is temporary and will last only until the hair is wet. Once the hair is wet the chemical (disulfide) bonds become active and the hair is once again curly.

There are several ways to approach quick-service for Black hair by using a blow-dryer. The hair can be completely styled using only the blow-dryer or it can be predried in preparation for press and curl, iron curling, or both.

BLOW-DRYING PRIOR TO PRESS AND CURL

Like any other hair care service, quick service styling begins by analyzing the hair to determine its natural texture and whether or not any damage exists. Most Black hair is fragile, especially if the hair has been chemically relaxed. Chemically treated hair is lacking in tensile strength and special care must be taken not to overstretch the hair during the blow-drying procedure.

SUGGESTED PROCEDURE

- After the hair has been cleansed and conditioned, begin preliminary drying. Use your fingers to lift and separate the strands as the hot air is directed into the hair. Follow this procedure until the excess moisture is removed. It is necessary that the hair remains in a "damp" condition.

- Begin to straighten the hair at the nape. Insert a wide-tooth, hard rubber or bone comb into a thin panel of hair. Move the comb slowly from the scalp toward the end, carefully following the comb movement with the warm air flow directed on the hair held by the comb. Continue to direct the air onto the top and bottom of each thin panel of hair from nape to the occipital bone. Force the hair in the direction the finished

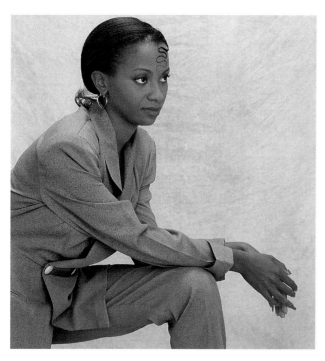

Dana, Hairstyle Technical #9

style will flow. Treat the hair as a fine, fragile fiber. Allow the comb to glide and direct the hair without excessive pulling or stretching.

- Roll the comb so the back is used to straighten and smooth as you let the length flow through the teeth.

- Work all the way around the perimeter, drying and directing, approximately three inches from the face frame toward the crown. Only when the perimeter is completed begin to blow-dry the interior.

- Part off easy-to-handle panels of hair. Work from the previously dried perimeter toward the crown. Move the air flow from scalp to hair ends. Be sure that each single panel of hair is thoroughly dry and straightened before moving on to another. If the hair is not thoroughly dry it will frizz and be very difficult to press.

- This procedure results in only a partial reduction of the existing tight curl. To further dry, direct, and smooth the hair, attach a more narrow attachment to the nozzle of the dryer and go back over the entire head using the same "direct and dry" procedure.

- A narrow nozzle concentrates the air flow, allowing you to apply more intense heat to resistant areas. For this part of the treatment replace the wide-tooth comb with a firm bristle brush. Be sure to keep the air flow moving so the hot air will not scorch the hair or burn the scalp.

- Continue to move the hair into a style pattern. Continue until the hair moves in the desired direction without resistance.

NOTE: The blow-drying procedure described may be followed by pressing, marcelling, or thermal iron curling. If, however, the hair is sufficiently styled by blow-drying alone, the service may stand alone.

AIR STYLING (BLOW-DRYING) LONG BLACK HAIR

- Long hair of any type requires more time, skill, and patience to blow-dry than short hair. Because most Black hair is fragile and easily overstretched, particular care must be taken.

- Begin the procedure by dividing clean, damp hair into four or more major sections. Twist the hair of each section in one direction until it forms one large, smooth roll from scalp to end. Coil the hair into a large knot and pin securely. This serves to somewhat stretch and prestraighten the hair while it's waiting to be air dried.

- Follow the same procedure as for short or mid-length hair.

NOTE: There is no mystery to blow-drying (air-forming) Black hair of any length if a basic technical procedure is followed and extreme caution is taken. Various blow-dryer attachments are manufactured specifically for use on Black hair. Each must be judged on its own merit.

Hair Coloring

REFERENCE CODE #105

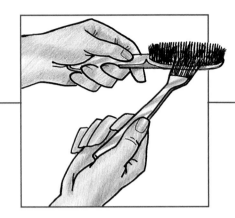

Color enhancement or even a complete color change can be an exciting option for clients of color, those whose hair color is naturally black.

Only a highly skilled color technician can effectively lift the natural hair color from jet black (levels 1, 2, or 3) to shades more than one or two levels lighter. The problem lies in the red and gold tones that must be neutralized before a lighter shade or toner can be applied.

The hair color of most African-Americans appears to be darkest black until it is examined in strong light. Then many shades are detectable. Most prominent are shades of black (levels 1 and 2) mixed with brown, red, and gold.

When a color product is mixed with a high-lift developer or any percentage of peroxide and applied to the hair, the blackest shades in the hair start to turn red, then gold, and finally yellow.

Many people of color have their naturally curly hair chemically relaxed. This strong chemical process weakens the hair, making it extremely porous, and as a result an addition chemical, such as bleach or tint, might cause breakage.

Black hair is best kept in color levels 1–3, with intensive surface color added for cosmetic illusion and shine as opposed to a penetrating tint.

Because Black hair is difficult to lift beyond levels of red, a nonoxidative hair-color product is often preferred over chemically activated products.

So-called nonpenetrating haircolor products are ideal for hair that has been chemically relaxed or straightened. Such products contain no lifting action, will not remove color from natural pigment, and will only deposit color that adds depth and tone to existing hair colors. It will also blend gray or faded hair. Many such products contain conditioning properties that are gentle on the hair.

Surface color (nonoxidative color) stains and seals the cuticle layer of the hair, making the surface smooth, and increasing the reflecting quality. It gives the appearance of color-glaze and ultra-shine.

Semi-permanent, surface coloring, and nonoxidizing, nonpenetrating color products are safe and effective on hair that is in good condition. If the hair is overporous or chemically damaged no color application will give effective, even coverage.

Just remember, prebleaching is not recommended for naturally Black hair. If an activated product is used, plan only to lift the natural color into levels of dark to medium brown.

Because porosity is the major factor in controlling color results, protein reconditioners are recommended before any color treatment.

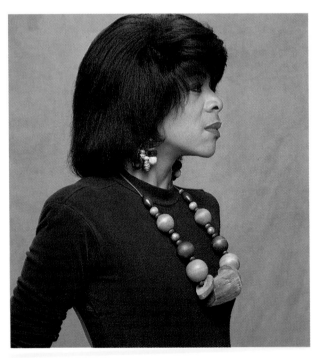

Dianne, Hairstyle Technical #1

Chemical Relaxing and Perming

REFERENCE CODE #106

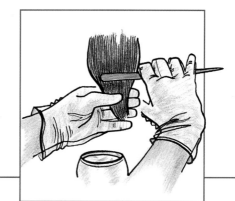

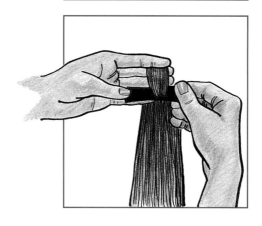

Chemical hair relaxing is the art of permanently restructuring excessively curly hair. It is a service most often required by Black clients whose hair has a genetic tendency to be tightly curled.

After a chemical relaxing service, the previously curly hair is left straight or with considerably less curl. It is also left in good condition if basic professional rules are followed.

Two types of chemicals are used to formulate relaxing products: sodium hydroxide and ammonium thioglycolate. Outlined are the most pertinent facts relating to both types.

SODIUM HYDROXIDE

Sodium hydroxide is a caustic-type relaxer with an alkaline pH of 10 and higher. This is the strongest chemical known to be used on human hair for any purpose. This type relaxer should only be applied by a salon professional who has extensive product knowledge and technical skill.

Sodium hydroxide has both a softening and swelling action on hair fibers. It penetrates the cortex layer of the hair, and breaks and unlocks the cross-bonds resulting in curl reduction. When the relaxer application is manipulated by a comb or with the hands, it is distributed throughout the strand and softens, relaxes, or straightens the hair.

When using sodium hydroxide, the application must be completed within a maximum period of eight minutes. To minimize possible chemical damage, the application should be left on the hair no longer than the time indicated by a strand test taken before the service. If the relaxer product is left on too long, the hair will become discolored and is apt to

break. There is a danger of completely dissolving the hair. Great care must be exercised at all times when using sodium hydroxide relaxer.

AMMONIUM THIOGLYCOLATE

This solution is somewhat milder than sodium hydroxide. The pH is approximately 9.2 compared to 10 and higher. It relaxes hair in much the same manner as sodium hydroxide but is not recommended for excessively curly hair. It simply will not remove as much of the curl. If the hair is wavy or curly, not kinky, ammonium thioglycolate quite effectively restructures the texture.

NEUTRALIZER

Neutralizer, or fixative, is also called a stabilizer and serves to stop the action of any chemical relaxer that may remain in the hair after rinsing. The neutralizer, most often in the form of shampoo, fixes or hardens the cross-bonds in their new position. Each manufacturer has specific instructions for the use of their product. Instructions should be followed carefully.

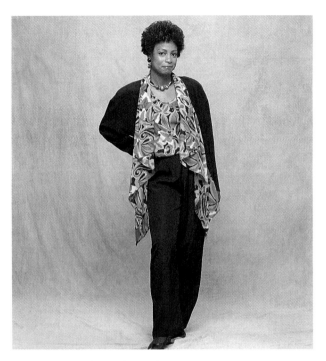

Mary, Hairstyle Technical #4

BASIC STEPS TO A SUCCESSFUL RELAXING SERVICE

CLIENT'S HAIR HISTORY Keep a record of each client that receives a chemical relaxer. Be sure to record that you have made a thorough scalp examination and given a strand test — both to the satisfaction of the client. If the hair is damaged or the scalp is in poor condition, don't execute the relaxing service until the problem has been corrected.

SCALP EXAMINATION Inspect carefully for the presence of lesions, scratches, or sores of any type. Part the hair into one-half inch sections with the index or middle finger. Take care not to scratch the scalp with a comb or your own fingernail.

STRAND TEST Three strand tests should be made prior to any relaxing service: finger test, pull test, relaxer test.

The Finger Test This test determines the degree of porosity. Hold a strand of hair between the thumb and index finger. Run the fingers from the end of the strand toward the scalp. If the hair ruffles, it is porous and capable of absorbing moisture.

The Pull Test This test determines the tensile strength. Tensile strength is also known as the elasticity of the hair. Curly hair will stretch about one-fifth of its normal length when dry without breaking. Hold a half dozen or so hairs firmly together and pull them gently. If the hair stretches and returns to its original length, it has elasticity and can withstand the relaxer process. If not, the hair must be conditioned until the reaction is favorable.

Relaxer Test Cut a hole in a piece of aluminum foil. Pull a few strands of hair through the hole and apply relaxer. Allow it to remain on the hair for two or three minutes. Remove with a piece of dry cotton. Test the degree of relaxation as related to the amount of time the relaxer was left on the hair. If the hair is not relaxed sufficiently, repeat the same process using a virgin strand and increase the timing. This test determines the amount of time needed for the degree of relaxation desired.

SECTIONING FOR THE RELAXER PRO-CEDURE Divide the hair into four sections — forehead to nape and ear to ear over the crest of the head. If the scalp is excessively moist put the client under a warm (not hot) dryer for a few minutes to correct the condition.

> Note: Depending on the product, a protective base may be required. Most relaxer products are "no-base" specified and no product other than the relaxer is required. However, if not, apply a protective base to the scalp at this time. In any case, apply protective cream on the facial area around the hairline.

Subdivide each of the four major sections into one-half inch partings and apply base freely to the entire scalp with the fingers. Do not rub. The base is actually "laid" on the scalp. Do not try to spread the base as body heat will insure complete distribution. Be sure the entire scalp and hairline are covered for protection.

Note: Before starting the application, check to be sure all materials necessary to give a relaxer service are properly assembled.

Checklist:
    Products
        Chemical relaxer
        Protective base (if required)
        Neutralizer/stabilizer
        Hair conditioner
    Equipment
        Towels
        Spatula
        Absorbent cotton
        Comb
        Timer
        Neck strip
    Styling Implements
        Rollers
        Hair blower
        Comb
        Clips/picks
        hair net
        Brush

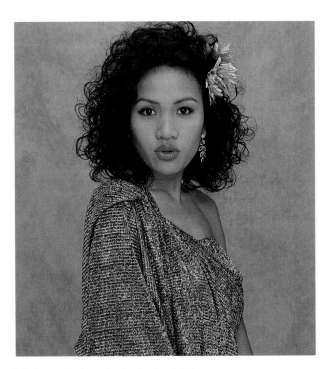

Vichett, Hairstyle Technical #5

APPLICATION PROCEDURE USING SODIUM HYDROXIDE

Divide the hair into four major sections. Less processing time is required at the scalp and on the ends, therefore, apply relaxer product to those areas last. Begin application at the back right section of the head. Subdivide the section into one-half inch horizontal panels. With a comb or spatula, scoop out a quantity of relaxing cream from the jar. Apply the relaxer starting one-half inch from the scalp and comb one inch of the ends. Leave more if the hair ends are severely damaged. Apply the relaxer cream to the underneath side of the same section. Fold the saturated strand out of the way straight over the curve of the head. Complete the back sections then move to the front. Do not apply relaxer to the hairline at this time.

When the relaxer has been applied to the entire head (in the procedure described) go back over the head applying relaxer cream to the one-half inch at the scalp, down to the ends, and around the hairline.

Never apply relaxer directly onto the scalp. Keep product on the hair, not on the scalp.

Either comb the cream down the strand or manipulate with the fingers to spread the relaxer product and aid relaxation. As the relaxer is spread, inspect the action by stretching the strand to determine how much curl is being removed from the hair. If the hair is relaxing too fast in any one area, the relaxer should be removed from the hair at the shampoo bowl immediately (only in that area). The process can be continued in other parts of the head. The relaxer should be combed onto the ends only at the very end of the procedure to prevent breakage. Very often, the ends will require some trimming in any case.

It is important to note here that the entire relaxer application must be completed in a maximum of eight minutes. Usually the processing time is from five to eight minutes as well. However, the total processing time is determined by the preprocess relaxer test.

When the hair is sufficiently relaxed, take the client to the shampoo bowl for rinsing, light shampoo/neutralizing, and conditioning. Handle wet, relaxed hair very gently during the styling process.

Thermal Irons/ Iron Curling

REFERENCE CODE #107

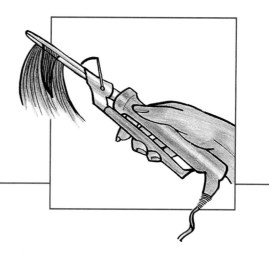

The method of creating waves in hair by using heated irons was introduced in 1875 by a French gentleman named Marcel Grateau. The method he introduced is still taught in beauty schools today as the best method of putting waves in dry hair. It is called *marcel waving*.

Today, the technique of temporarily changing hair structure by the use of heat on dry hair is called Thermal Waving or Iron Curling. Thermal waving can best be described as the art of imparting waves and/or curls to straight or pressed hair by means of heated, cylindrical irons and a special manipulative technique.

Knowledge, skill, and lots of practice are required to master the art of thermal waving. If you are totally unfamiliar with the use of curling irons, start initial practice using cold irons on a strand of hair before ever trying it with heated irons.

You were probably introduced to marcel irons during your basic cosmetology course in a class identified as Thermal Curling. Marcel irons, the type heated in ovens, are not widely used in today's modern salons. But there's no better way to master the art of "iron curling" of any type, than manipulating the irons and reviewing the technique and basic procedure before actually performing the service.

MANIPULATIVE PROCEDURE (HANDLING THE IRON)

Use a cold iron for practice. Hold the closed irons with the groove on the bottom of the irons. Using only one hand, slowly turn the irons one-half turn away from you, bringing the groove to the top of the irons. Now, still using only one hand, turn the irons another quarter turn, bringing the groove to rest vertically on the opposite side from where you are standing. Complete the turn, bringing the groove to rest on the bottom, the position from which you started. You have executed one complete turn with the irons closed.

Now repeat the routine, opening the irons (holding the groove away from the barrel) each time you make a quarter turn.

When you have mastered the rotating technique it is time to learn the waving procedure.

MARCEL WAVE (practice with cold iron)

1. For practice purposes start at a side part on the light side. You will be working with a panel of hair approximately two inches wide.

2. Make a horizontal part across the two-inch panel of hair approximately two inches from the style part. Insert the hair in the irons with the barrel on top. The groove is on the bottom, facing upward.

3. Open the irons slightly and make one-half turn away from you. That, technically speaking, is "forward" turn.

4. Now with the irons closed, turn backward (toward yourself) to the original position. Open the irons slightly, separating the barrel from the groove, and slide them down the strand of hair one inch, then close the irons.

5. Turn the irons one full turn away from yourself (forward turn).

6. Now, with the irons closed turn one full turn in the opposite direction, back to the original position.

7. Release the hair from the irons. You have completed a practice marcel waving technique.

YOU ARE READY TO EXECUTE A WAVE USING HEATED IRONS

Before beginning to wave, comb the hair in a semi-shaping — "C" shaping — half a finger wave.

1. Using a hard rubber styling comb, pick up a strand of hair about two inches in width. Insert the irons into the hair with the groove facing upward (on the bottom). The panel of hair is now between the groove and the barrel of the irons.

2. Close the irons and turn them about one-quarter turn forward (away from you). At the same time, draw the hair with the irons about one-quarter inch to the left. Simultaneously direct the hair about one-quarter inch to the right with the comb. (The comb is in your left hand at all times.)

3. Now make one full forward turn of the irons (away from you). Be sure to keep the hair uniform with the comb. The hair has a tendency to roll at a slight slant on the groove of the iron. Hold that position for a few seconds to allow the hair to become sufficiently heated throughout the panel of hair being waved.

4. At this time reverse the movement by unrolling the hair from the irons, bringing it back into its first resting position. (When the movement is completed, the comb will be resting slightly away from the irons.)

5. Open the irons with the little finger and place the irons just below the ridge of the wave by swinging the slightly open irons toward you and then closing them. The outside edge of the groove will be directly underneath the ridge just created by the inner edge of the groove.

6. Hold the irons in place and use the comb to direct the hair toward the left about one inch. This movement forms the hair into a half circle.

7. Keep the irons closed and roll them one-half turn forward (away from you). As you make this movement keep the comb perfectly still and in the same position.

8. Slightly open the irons (called a loose grip) and slide the irons down the strand of hair about one inch.

The comb and irons are in a position to make the second ridge and the beginning of a wave going to the right. Manipulate all the movements executed for the previous wave going to the left with one exception: the hair is directed opposite to that of a wave going to the left.

After the first two-inch panel of hair is completely waved from scalp to ends, the next adjacent panel should be waved to match each movement perfectly.

The same basic technique is followed to wave each succeeding panel of hair. However, while picking up the unwaved hair in the comb, a small section of the formerly waved strand must be included as a guide to the formation of the new wave. Be sure the comb and iron movements are the same as in the first strand of hair, otherwise the waves will not match.

Repeat the procedure as many times as it takes to wave the entire head or any portion you want waved.

> NOTE: When thermal waving, use the same basic patterns used in wet finger waving.

SHADOW THERMAL WAVING

Shadow thermal waving is nothing more than making waves without ridges on the surface of the hair. The underneath hair and that next to the scalp is not waved.

All manipulations should be practiced until an entire head of hair can be waved in a very short amount of time.

When the waving is finished the hair may be combed to give it a softer look, and a holding spray used if necessary.

Hair Pressing

REFERENCE CODE #108

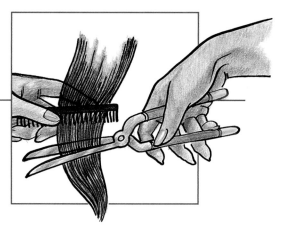

Hair pressing is also called "silking." It is the art of temporarily straightening excessively curly hair.

Hair pressing is done by using a heated, metal comb having a barrel back. The comb is heated to a temperature suitable to the type hair that is being straightened then combed through the hair. The back (barrel) of the comb actually does the straightening. The hair is combed and stretched into a straight condition.

The hair will remain in that straight condition until it is wet. Although the hair has been temporarily straightened, it has not been chemically restructured, and unlike hair that has been chemically relaxed, it will revert to its curly state when exposed to moisture.

The pressing comb is ideal for Black women and men who do not want their hair chemically treated, but desire straighter hair for better control and the pleasure of wearing modern hairstyles.

There are several methods of hair pressing. The amount of curl you wish to remove determines the type of pressing that is done. If all the curl is to be removed from the hair, the procedure calls for a hard press. If three-fourths of the curl is to be removed, the method used is called a medium press. If you wish to remove only half of the curl, the most effective method is called a soft press. Once the excess curl is removed by any one of the methods, the hair is usually curled with a thermal (curling) iron to give it movement and direction.

Like any other service on Black hair, hair pressing requires a thorough analysis of the hair and scalp before beginning the service. The condition of the hair will help determine the amount of heat and pressure that can safely be used. If the hair is dry and porous, the heat and pressure needed to straighten it must be reduced. Hair that has been tinted or light-ened also requires special attention. Oily hair is usually less porous and requires more heat and pressure to straighten.

PRESSING OIL OR CREAM

The application of pressing oil or cream prior to a hair pressing treatment can help protect the hair. Those products help to soften the hair, condition, prevent burning or scorching, prevent breakage and add shine. No product, of course, takes the place of proper hair analysis, proper type press, and skill in manipulating the pressing comb.

The pressing comb may also be used between salon visits to straighten hair around the face or in areas where it may have reverted to its natural state.

STANDARD PROCEDURE FOR A SOFT PRESS

The soft press procedure removes the least amount of natural curl of any of the pressing procedures. Each press soft, medium, and hard, is executed by following the same basic steps listed below (with only slight changes for each).

- Examine the scalp and analyze the hair.
- Shampoo, rinse, and towel dry the hair.
- Apply a small amount of pressing oil or cream and work it throughout the damp hair, then complete the drying process.
- Start heating the pressing combs.
- Divide the hair into easy-to-handle sections and clip in place.
- Remove tangles from one of the back sections in preparation for pressing.

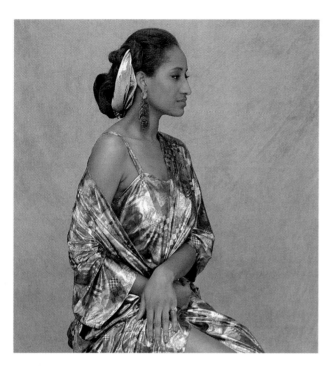

Diedra, Hairstyle Technical #7

- Test the temperature of the pressing comb on white tissue paper. If the paper discolors allow the comb to cool.
- Hold the hair straight out from the head. Insert the teeth of the comb on top of the strand, as near the scalp as possible without touching the scalp.
- Rotate the teeth of the comb away from the head so the back rod (barrel) of the comb makes contact with the hair. The back of the comb is the part that does the straightening.
- Hold the hair strand firmly against the comb and slowly draw the comb through the entire hair strand. Maintain constant pressure on the comb.
- Now insert the teeth of the comb on the underside of the same strand, as near the scalp as possible, and repeat the procedure used on top of the strand. This time the teeth of the comb will be pointed up.

- Repeat the pressing procedure on top and/or underneath as many times as necessary to straighten the hair.
- Part out a one-fourth inch panel of hair immediately above the pressed strand and repeat the pressing procedure.
- Continue to part the hair into one-fourth inch panels and use the same pressing procedure until all the hair on the head has been pressed.

HARD PRESS

A hard press is exactly like the soft press except the entire procedure is repeated. It is also referred to as a *double press*.

A hard press is recommended only when the results of a soft press are not satisfactory. After the hair has cooled from the first press, add pressing oil (sparingly) and work it through the hair. Repeat the exact pressing procedure.

A hard press is seldom necessary if you carefully press each strand over and over until it is perfectly straight during the first press. It is more time consuming to do it twice than it is to do it right the first press.

PRESS TOUCH-UP

This means only that certain sections of the hair are repressed when the hair begins to revert to its curly state due to perspiration or dampness. The procedure is the same as the initial press (omitting the shampoo). Ordinarily, a press touch-up is done only around the hairline.

PRECAUTIONS

The most obvious precaution is to not burn the client nor scorch the hair. Extreme care must be taken at all times when using hot implements.

When pressing very short hair use a cool iron near the hairline.

When pressing coarse hair be sure the pressing sections are very narrow, that the comb is sufficiently hot, and that enough pressure is given so the hair remains in a straightened condition.

Hot Combing

REFERENCE CODE #109

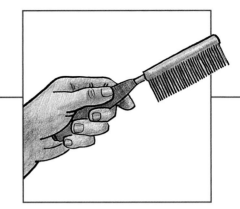

The hot comb is not a preferred tool for altering the texture of Black hair in its natural state. It is often referred to as a "touch-up" or "maintenance" device. It is most effective on Black hair that has been chemically relaxed.

It is an effective tool to create instant volume, indentation, waves, or curls. A hot cob is actually a combination of a comb, blow dryer, and curling iron. The hair is guided through the teeth of the comb and the hair is directed as desired.

When using a hot comb, small sections of hair are used at a time to allow air from the tool to penetrate through each section, drying and molding the hair quickly.

The hot comb should always be used on freshly shampooed hair. The length of time required to dry and curl or wave the hair depends on the thickness and the length of hair being serviced.

If you are proficient in the art of finger waving, or positioning rollers in wet hair for a desired pattern, using the hot comb is not unlike those basic procedures. All the fundamental rules apply. The primary difference is that you hold the styling comb in the left hand and the hot comb in the right. It is an easy technique to learn. Like all other hairstyling skills, it requires practice.

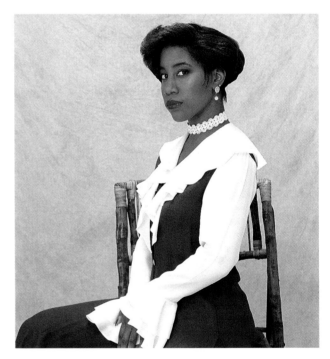

Christine, Hairstyle Technical #8

Specialty Hair Styling: Hair Extension

REFERENCE CODE #110

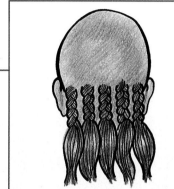

Hair extension is the art of adding length and/or volume to human hair growing on the head. This is done by one of several techniques — weaving or bonding being the most popular.

Weaving is the technique most often used in today's modern salons. Hair can be added for volume where the hair is sparse or on balding areas. It is used as well for aesthetic purposes to give instant length to short hair, to add length and volume to hair that has breakage caused by chemical treatments, or simply to create dramatic or exotic hairstyles.

Many Black celebrities wear hair-weaves — most notably Diana Ross and Whitney Houston. However, hair weaving is not used exclusively by Black clients. Many Caucasian clients take advantage of instant length and unusual glamour.

An added advantage of hair weaving is that it can be removed fairly easy with no damage to the natural hair growth. For that reason it is used often to camouflage breakage while the hair grows back to a healthy state.

Depending on the technique used and the extent of the weave, the time it takes to complete a weave is relatively short. The service is considered highly specialized and a hair designer must have special training in order to weave hair properly.

There is a sophisticated tool manufactured for the purpose of hair weaving. However, most hair-weave artists use a technique that requires a minimum number of tools but a lot of know-how.

When a weave is properly executed, the service is fast, and there are no visible lumps or bumps caused by uneven attachments.

NECESSARY TOOLS

(to be assembled before beginning the service)

- Two or more weaving needles
- Plenty of strong nylon weaving thread (the same color as the hair)
- Appropriate human or synthetic hair (wefts) (Human hair is preferred. If synthetic hair is used it must be of the highest quality fabric.)

PREPARATION PRIOR TO SERVICE

First, human hair that has been sewn into "wefts" is perfectly matched to the client's own hair.

TEXTURE
The exact amount of curl as that of the client's own hair.

LENGTH
A predetermined length based on the desired finished style and practicality.

COLOR
The exact color is most desirable and the least detectable, however, highlights can be added as long as shades are compatible. The object is to create a style that has no visible artificiality.

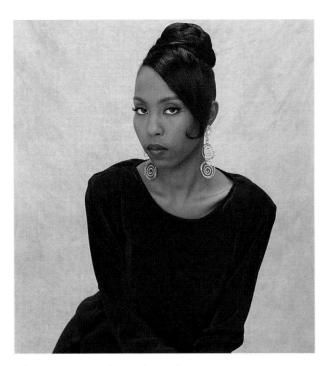

Theresa, Hairstyle Technical #11

SUGGESTED PROCEDURE

This is a procedure most often used if the purpose of the "extension" service is to add length.

- First, starting about three inches above the nape, divide the hair into several horizontal sections, extending completely around the head, from ear to ear. End each about one inch behind the facial hairline.

> **Note:** The number of sections and the space between each depends on how much hair you wish to add and the density of the natural hair. Most often three to five sections is sufficient to make a luxuriant hairstyle.

- When the lower crown is reached, continue to divide the hair into sections over the crest (the natural curve) of the head. Each section should end well behind the natural hairline.
- Measure and cut the length of the weft to the exact area it will be sewn. It is desirable to have one string of wefted hair extend from one side of the head to the other. Each time you start a new weft it requires reinforcement, making it more difficult to obtain a smooth base.
- Start at the lowest horizontal section at one outer edge or the other. (This often depends on whether you are right- or left-handed — either is correct.) Part a horizontal panel of hair using one side of the sectional part, about one-half inch wide. Begin twisting the hair very close to the head. Use the threaded needle to make a stitch around the twisted hair much like a "buttonhole stitch." When the one-half inch panel has been twisted and sewn securely from one end of the section to the other, without breaking the thread, start attaching the weft to the twisted and sewn panel. Secure the beginning and the end of each section very well. Leave a tail of extra thread about two inches long at each end when clipping.
- Let the hair down over the initial weft and proceed to the next highest section, working toward the crown. Repeat the procedure used on the initial weave.
- Continue to repeat the process, one section at a time until a weft has been attached to each section.

A WORD OF CAUTION

Don't be tempted to make the hair too full on the top. Make wide sections and hair can be added more easily than it can be removed.

MAINTENANCE

When the hair grows, the weaves will need to be tightened. Inasmuch as the hair grows one-half inch a month, it will be some time before any repair will be needed.

The hair may be shampooed just as if it all was growing from the scalp. The only precaution is that care should be taken not to tangle it during the cleansing process.

The wefts can be removed by simply clipping the nylon thread, being especially careful not to clip any of the natural hair. The weft may be used repeatedly.

The original color of the hair wefts may fade over a period of time. If the extensions are made of human hair it will accept a hair color product. Synthetic fibers cannot be colored with any of the human hair color products. Great care must be taken when refreshing the color of hair wefts. Use a nonperoxide product for best results. Keep in mind that color developers (peroxide) act to lift color from the hair before depositing color pigments. Hair wefts need only "color deposit."

The price of an extension service (weaving) varies. As usual the basic fee includes the time spent on the service and the products used. Hair wefts (especially human hair) can be quite expensive, and the reputation and the skill of the technician makes a great deal of difference.

HAIR WEAVE ALTERNATIVE TECHNIQUE

BRAID/CORN ROW ATTACHMENT

A common technique used for hair extension is to follow the same basic parting procedure and preparation as that outlined for the weaving technique. Instead of twisting, rolling, and stitching the base panel of hair, braid it into a very fine corn row. Then attach the weft to the corn row. This technique may leave a higher ridge at the connection point than the twisting technique.

BONDING ATTACHMENT

Bonding is actually a very different service, but nevertheless comes under the subject of hair extension.

The tools you need:
A glue gun (dispenser)
A heating iron/device
Hair swatches (unattached to a weft)

The natural hair, where additional length is to be added, is divided into narrow blocks approximately one inch by one inch square. Several blocks may be separated in advance of the service and held with small clips.

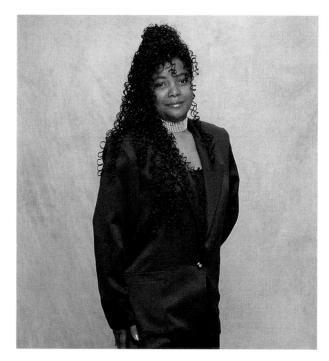

Betty, Hairstyle Technical #12

Comb the selected strands smooth, overlap the ends of a swatch of hair the same thickness as the natural hair, apply warm glue to both sides, and hold them firmly until they are fused. If there's any doubt about the security of the attachment, additional heat may be added using a warm flat iron in which you encase both pieces.

This procedure is repeated in any and all areas you wish to add hair by the bonding technique. This is a useful technique when hair damage is being repaired around the hairline. The attachment is very flat and not easily detected.

The bonded swatches can easily be removed by once again applying heat to the bonded area and then gently detaching the artificial strand. The hair ends containing the glue substance must be cut off. If they have been skillfully attached, the glue only extends about a half inch on the ends of both the natural hair and the added swatch.

Part II

HAIRSTYLE TECHNICALS

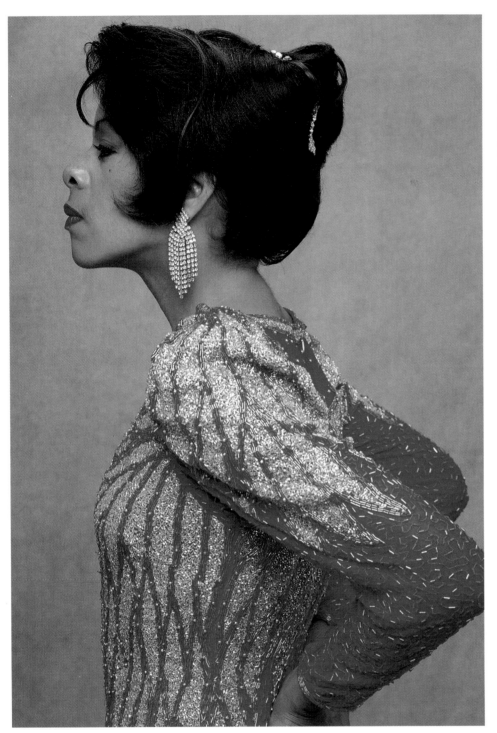

Style is the harmonious blending of one's most promi-nent qualities… physical features and personality.

Dianne

SERVICES

SEMI-PERMINENT HAIRCOLOR
HAIR CUTTING
WET SET

TECHNICAL REFERENCE NUMBER 103, 105

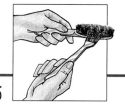
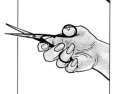
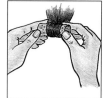

Typical of all professional salon clients, Dianne wants hair that looks healthy and great, that's contemporary in design, and is easily maintained. A nonoxidizing, semi-permanent color with just a touch of dramatic highlight quickly and effectively provides a soft, becoming corona of color and sheen.

Minimal shaping to remove damaged and stringy ends allows the hair to respond to a wet set that can be combed into a variety of smart styles. It can be worn airy and casual or sleek and exotic to meet the challenge posed by an active lifestyle.

To service your Black clientele to their best advantage, it is important to realize fashionable ladies all have at least one thing in common — they want to look their personal best.

Because we live in a very sophisticated society, your clients will seldom come to you having hair in a natural condition — hair that has not been chemically treated in one of several ways. Make a careful analysis, taking all factors into consideration and give her your best professional advice.

Dianne's personal hair analysis is permanently recorded.

DIANNE

HAIR ANALYSIS

Natural Texture: Wave ☐   Curl ☐   Kink ☑

Previous Chemical Service: Relaxed ☑   Straightened ☐   Colored ☐

Code:	1	2	3	4	5	6	7	8	9	10	
Porosity			✓								
Elasticity				✓							
Density				✓							
Coarseness					✓						
Hair Condition		✓									
Scalp Condition	✓										
Existing Gray		✓									

Technical Reference Number	103	105		

Code based on a scale numbered 1–10

#1 = Good/Average

#10 = Poor/Abnormal

SERVICES RECOMMENDED

SEMI-PERMANENT (NON OXIDIZING) HAIRCOLOR

Used to provide shine, camouflage existing gray, or add subtle color interest.

HAIR SHAPING

Done to balance uneven lengths throughout and to remove stringy, damaged ends.

WET ROLLER SET

Used to offer maximum control or create directional design.

PROCEDURE

SEMI-PERMANENT HAIRCOLOR (WITH DIMENSIONAL ACCENT)

Note: Semi-permanent hair color cannot be used to lift color from the hair. Instead it penetrates deep into the hair strand and departs rich, vibrant shades equal or darker than the natural hair color. Color pigments may be added for special effects. The use of "hair painting" prior to the color application lends a surprisingly dramatic effect.

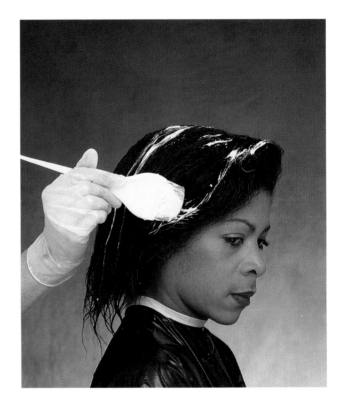

1 Mix high-lift powder bleach with thirty volume peroxide to a thin paste consistency. Comb the hair in the direction it will flow when styled. Use the side of a tint applicator brush to paint thin lines where you wish highlighted accents.

2 Allow the bleach to remain on the hair only until it lifts the natural color no more than two levels. Remove the bleach before it decolorizes the hair into an orange level. Lightly shampoo the bleach from the hair and gently towel dry to remove excess moisture.

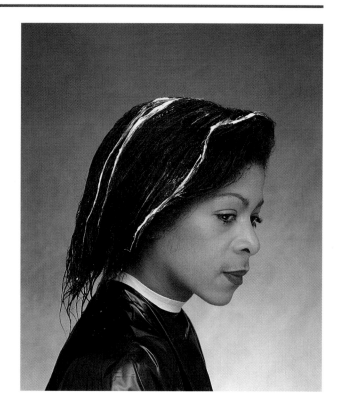

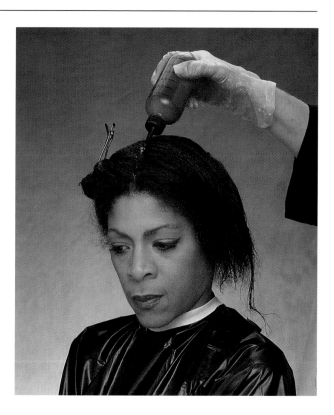

3 Divide the hair into four equal sections. Start in the center crown and apply tint to narrow horizontal sections.

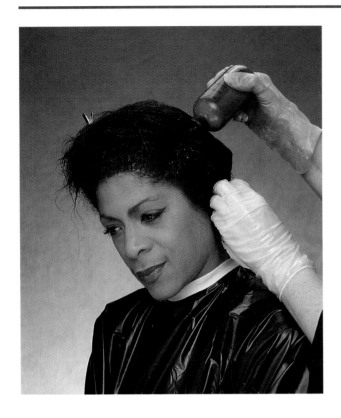

4 Apply tint systematically until all sections are thoroughly saturated.

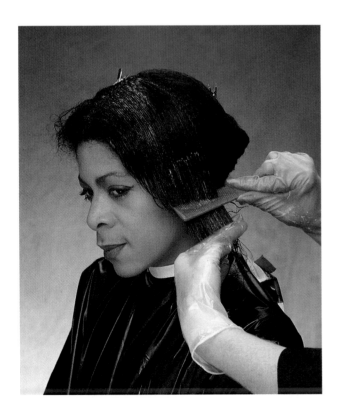

5 Use a wide-tooth tint comb to pull the tint from the scalp through the ends.

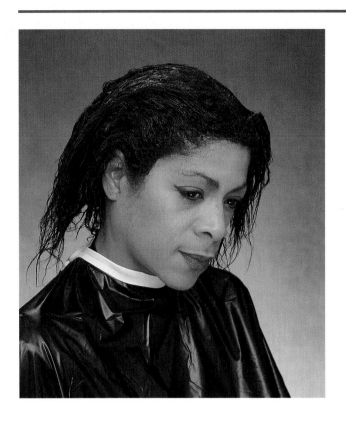

6 When the tint has been combed through, use your gloved hands to gently mulch the tint to be sure all hair is sufficiently covered with tint.

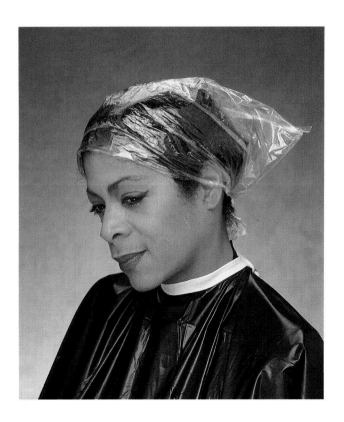

7 Cover the hair with a plastic cap. Carefully secure the cap at the back so it will not interfere with the tint process. Follow manufacturer's instructions as to whether or not it should be placed under heat during the processing time.

Note: When processing is complete, lightly shampoo the hair, rinse thoroughly, and condition as necessary. Towel dry the hair and blow it straight in preparation for shaping.

HAIR SHAPING

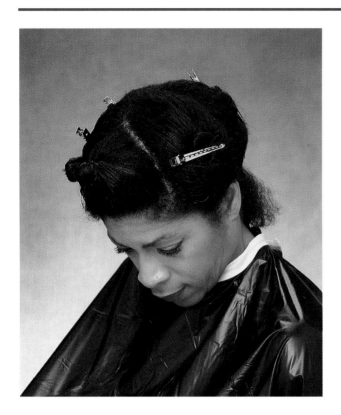

8 Divide the hair into triangular sections so the hair can be let down into its natural fall.

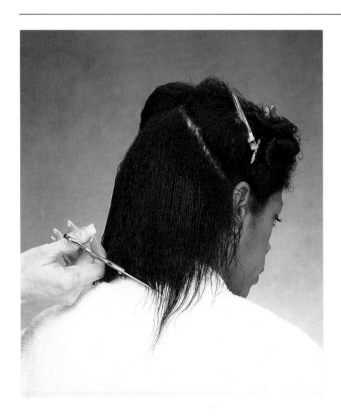

9 Start in the center back and trim all loose ends straight across. (The client is letting the hair grow into a longer bob.)

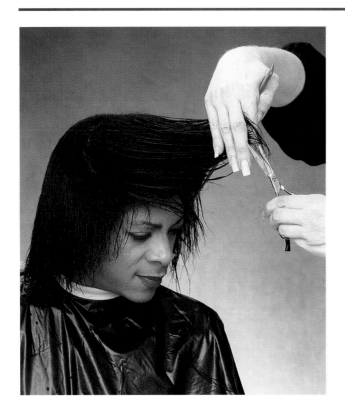

10 No layering is desired in the back area. For that reason hold all hair in the front triangle as far forward as possible. Remove only the stringy ends so the hair will be stronger in its continued growth.

WET ROLLER SET

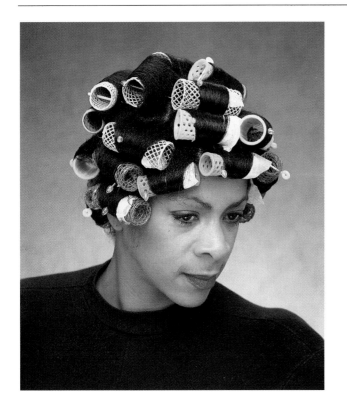

11 Use large diameter mesh rollers and hair picks, as opposed to hair clips, for securing each roller. Hair clips sometimes cause damage to extremely fragile hair, especially after a chemical service.

12 Start in the center crown and position on-base rollers directed toward the hairline in each area of the head. The diameter of each roller should be as large as possible allowing only one and one-half turn of the hair on the roller.

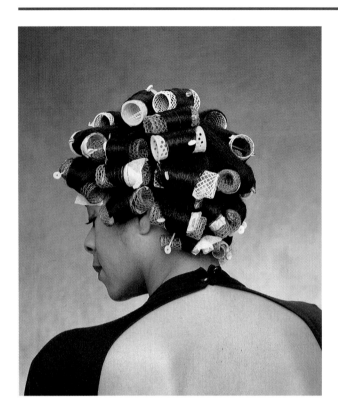

13 Wrap each rod with sufficient tension to keep the hair smooth during the drying process. Avoid excess tension and take care not to scrape the scalp when placing the picks.

Note: Place the client under a medium-hot hooded dryer and allow plenty of time for the hair to become free of all moisture. Never attempt to comb or brush Black hair that is not completely dry. The hair is ready now to be combed and brushed into a variety of attractive style options.

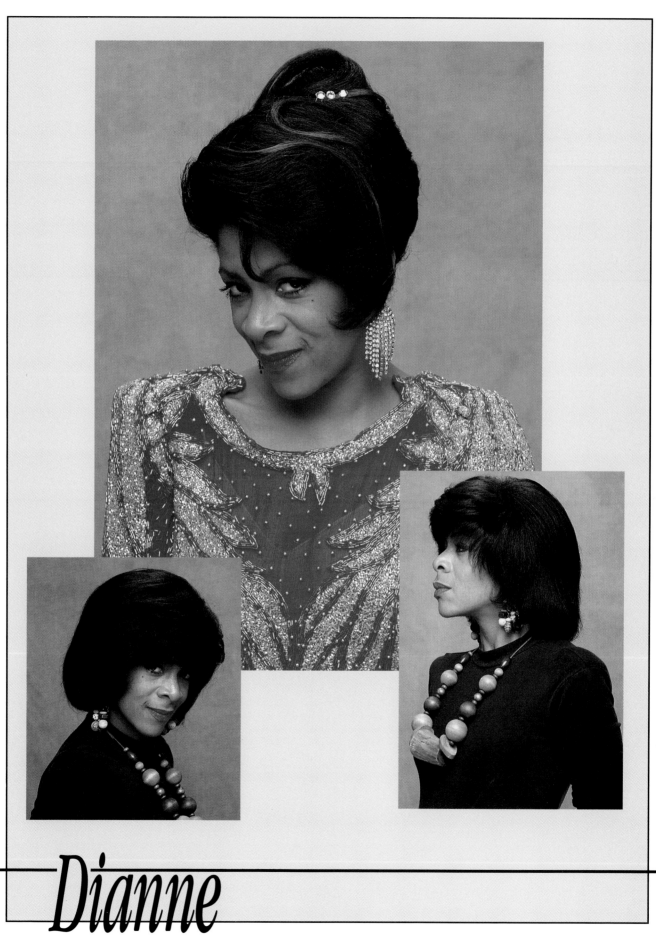

Dianne

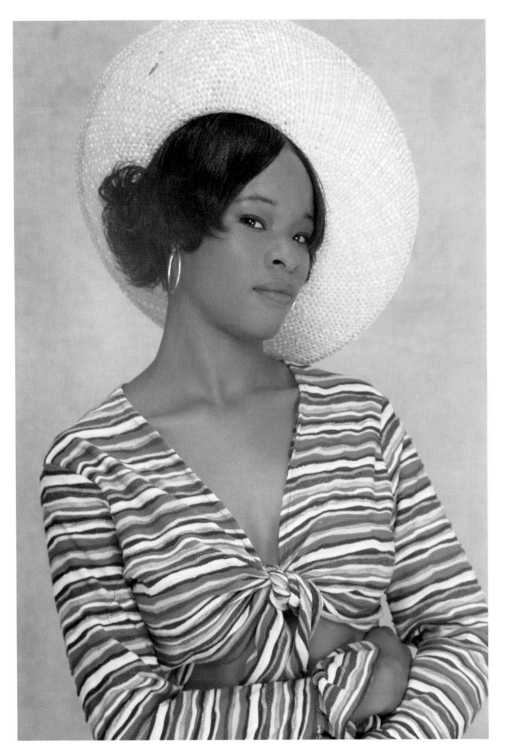

A daptability is more than a frame that flatters the face — it is complete only when you capture the essence of one's inner self.

No. 2 *Karen*

SERVICES

CUTTING DRY HAIR

TECHNICAL REFERENCE NUMBER 103

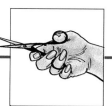

The term "full service salon" certainly applies to those professional establishments offering hair care and styling options to Black clients. It seems there is no so-called standard procedure that applies to everyone. Like any other community, the Black community is a diversified group whose demands and needs are as unique as each individual.

Karen prefers to keep much of her own curl and incorporate it into a hairstyle that primarily requires only that the length and form be trendy and easily maintained.

Like many busy career clients she pops into the salon for a trim (professional sculpting) on her dry hair, so all she has to do is rush back to her office looking her best.

This client regularly applies styling cream (grease) to her hair for control, definition of curl, and shine. It looks great but is a little tricky to handle when cutting. It is suggested that a damp towel be used to remove excess oil before starting the service.

The technical reason for cutting extra curly hair when it is dry: it enables the designer to cut to the exact desired length without fear of shrinkage. When Black hair is cut in a wet state the designer must keep in mind that the hair when dried will be one-fifth or more shorter than it appears when wet. For that reason dry-hair cutting can be a very valuable service to both client and salon professional.

When the hair was analyzed, which is always done even if no chemical service is anticipated, these were the findings. The client's hair analysis should become a permanent record and be updated at each visit. It is a great way to build repeat services. The client learns to trust your professional system and judgment.

KAREN

HAIR ANALYSIS

Natural Texture: Wave ☐ Curl ☑ Kink ☐

Previous Chemical Service: Relaxed ☑ Straightened ☐ Colored ☐

Code:	1	2	3	4	5	6	7	8	9	10	
Porosity					✓						
Elasticity					✓						
Density			✓								
Coarseness			✓								
Hair Condition					✓						
Scalp Condition	✓										
Existing Gray	○										

Technical Reference Number **103**

Code based on a scale number 1–10

#1 = Good/Average

#10 = Poor/Abnormal

SERVICE RECOMMENDED

As this is a first visit, the client is given the exact service that she requested — a dry cut. As a special treat and introduction to the salon, the designer suggested various ways Karen's hair might be worn.

PROCEDURE

Either use a cutting cape or a model-tube when cutting dry hair. Bare shoulders allow you to more accurately judge the perimeter lengths as related to neck and shoulders.

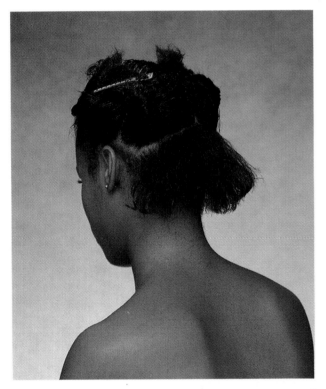

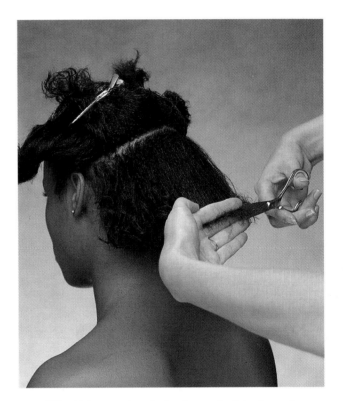

1 Divide the hair into sections for ease of handling. Establish the hanging length at center nape. Only hold the hair with enough tension for control. Excess tension in different areas of the head will result in the hair springing into uneven lengths.

2 Comb the hair down and away from the head at a forty-five degree angle to make sure the length is correct.

3 Direct the hair from behind each ear toward the center and cut it even with the original hanging guide.

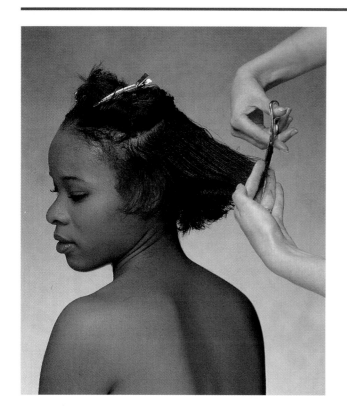

4 From this point the hair is let down in two-inch horizontal panels, held forty-five degrees from the head form, and cut even with the previously cut guide. This method results in a slight graduation from nape to center back.

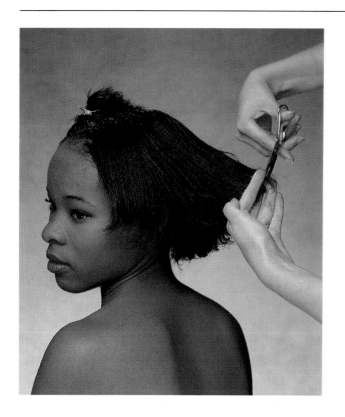

5 Work from side to side blending the side lengths with those of the back. Remember to comb, hold, and cut each section in the area in which it falls naturally. (Cutting to the natural fall of the hair is more difficult on curly hair, especially if it has styling cream applied that tends to keep it from falling naturally onto the head form.)

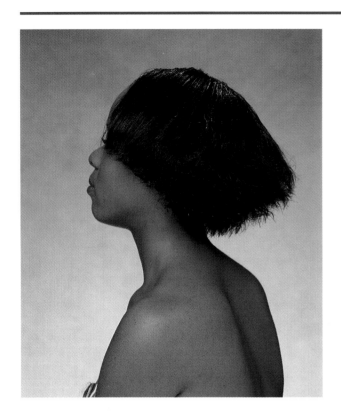

6 Continue the same cutting procedure until all the hair has been shortened and blended throughout.

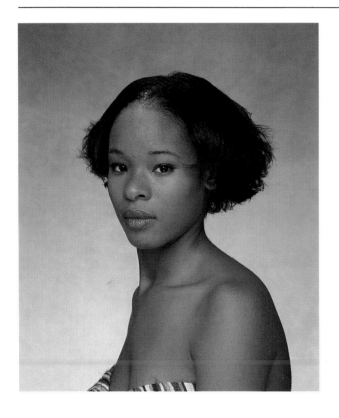

7 Part the hair in the center and shape the hanging length on each side from eye level to the established length behind each ear.

8 Styling of the bangs is optional. Karen wants her hair to grow longer in the front so the frontal area is divided evenly from a center part and blended with each side.

FINISHED STYLES

This hairstyle is adaptable to a variety of looks. The hair can be piled onto the top of the head and a scarf worn. It looks great worn just "as is," bringing down a fringe onto the forehead. A beach hat looks great, or add a multi-colored hair swatch to one side, cover it with a saucy hat, and voilà! A grunge look!

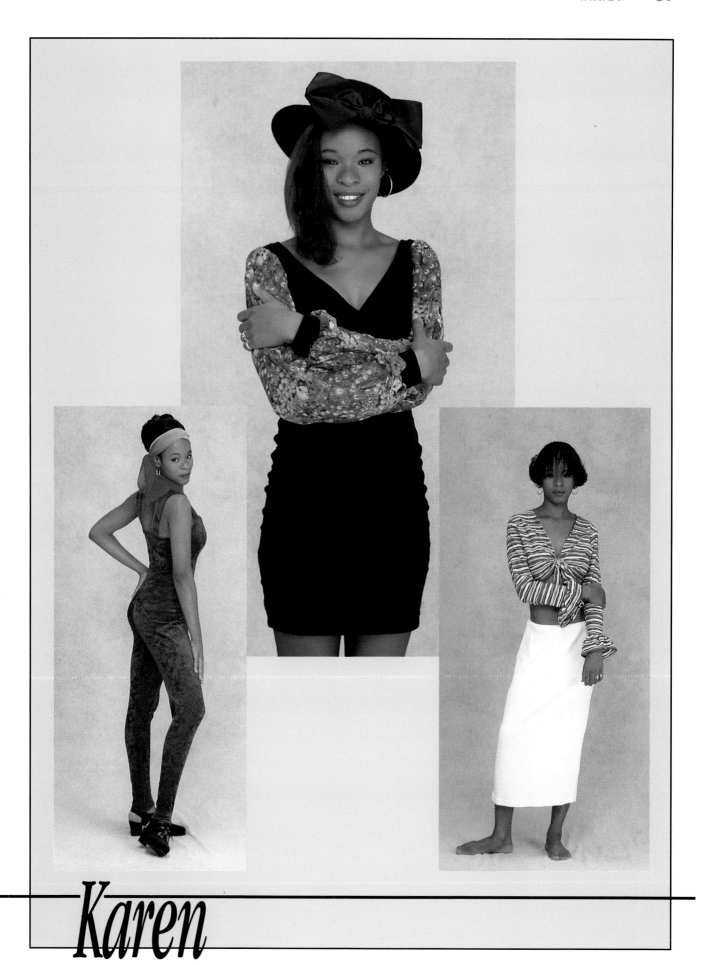

Karen

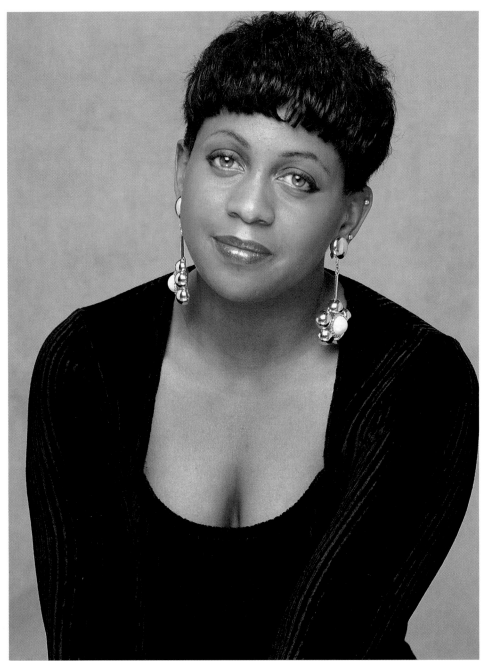

A hairstyle must complement the attitude of the wearer and reinforce her feeling of confidence.

No. 3 *Julie*

SERVICES

VIRGIN TINT
SEMI-PERMANENT COLOR

TECHNICAL REFERENCE NUMBER 105

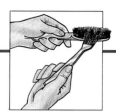

Whether you're adding a dash of color, covering gray, or creating something truly dramatic, the more you know about the different color processes and techniques, the more effective you will be as a color technician.

Permanent haircolor using full-strength developer is not ordinarily suitable to Black hair. The hair is, by nature, more porous and often more easily damaged than hair of the average white person.

For that reason, products used for virgin tints are carefully selected for their gentle qualities. This means either lower volume or no peroxide and no ammonia. The gentler the product, the less penetration into the hair shaft, resulting in a color that lasts longer than color conditioners but less than permanent color.

Hair of an African-American male or female has the same qualities. It stands to reason semi-permanent color that penetrates a bit deeper and lasts a little longer would be the product of choice for all short Black hair.

Analyze the hair and scalp carefully before any chemical service. A strand test is strongly recommended before all virgin tints.

Julie's personal analysis becomes a permanent record.

JULIE

HAIR ANALYSIS

Natural Texture: Wave ☐   Curl ☐   Kink ☑

Previous Chemical Service: Relaxed ☑   Straightened ☐   Colored ☐

Code:	1	2	3	4	5	6	7	8	9	10	
Porosity		✓									
Elasticity		✓									
Density				✓							
Coarseness			✓								
Hair Condition		✓									
Scalp Condition	✓										
Existing Gray		✓									

Technical Reference Number		**105**				

Code based on a scale number 1–10

#1 = Good/Average

#10 = Poor/Abnormal

SERVICE RECOMMENDED

The hair has been previously relaxed; a period of two weeks has lapsed. A protein conditioner was applied one week ago. The hair being in good conditon will undoubtedly take a semi-permanent hair color to best advantage.

PROCEDURE

Shampoo and condition the hair so it is soft and pliable. Avoid rubbing the scalp. Remove excess moisture with an absorbent towel leaving the hair slightly damp. The cuticle remains open in damp hair allowing the color molecules to penetrate the hair shaft more easily.

1 Mix the tint formula in a nonmetallic container and use a firm tint brush for the application. Wear gloves to prevent staining your fingernails. A virgin semi-permanent tint application may start in any one of four sections. Here it is started in the front area.

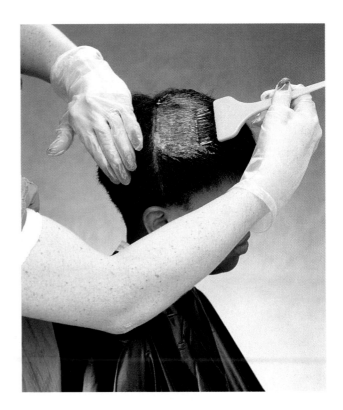

2 Use long stokes to first outline the entire section.

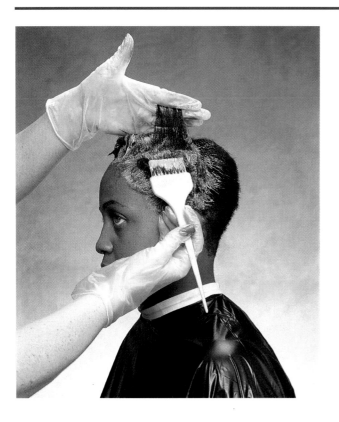

3 Subdivide the section by making narrow, horizontal partings. Apply a generous amount of tint to each side of the panel.

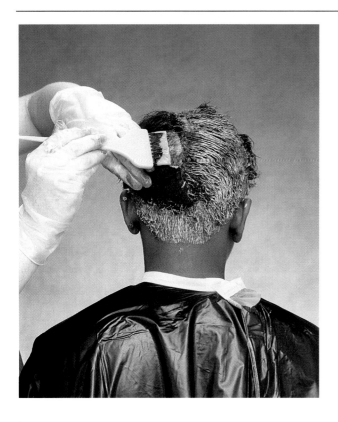

4 Continue the initial application procedure until each of the four sections are completely saturated.

5 Using your gloved hand and a wide-tooth tint comb distribute the tint throughout and allow it to process. Processing requirements vary for different tint products. Best results can be obtained by following the manufacturer's instructions.

Note: When tint has reached its fullest color potential, shampoo and condition the hair. The hair may be styled by any method but it is best to avoid very hot curling or blowing instruments immediately following a chemical process. The hair is easily damaged by excess heat.

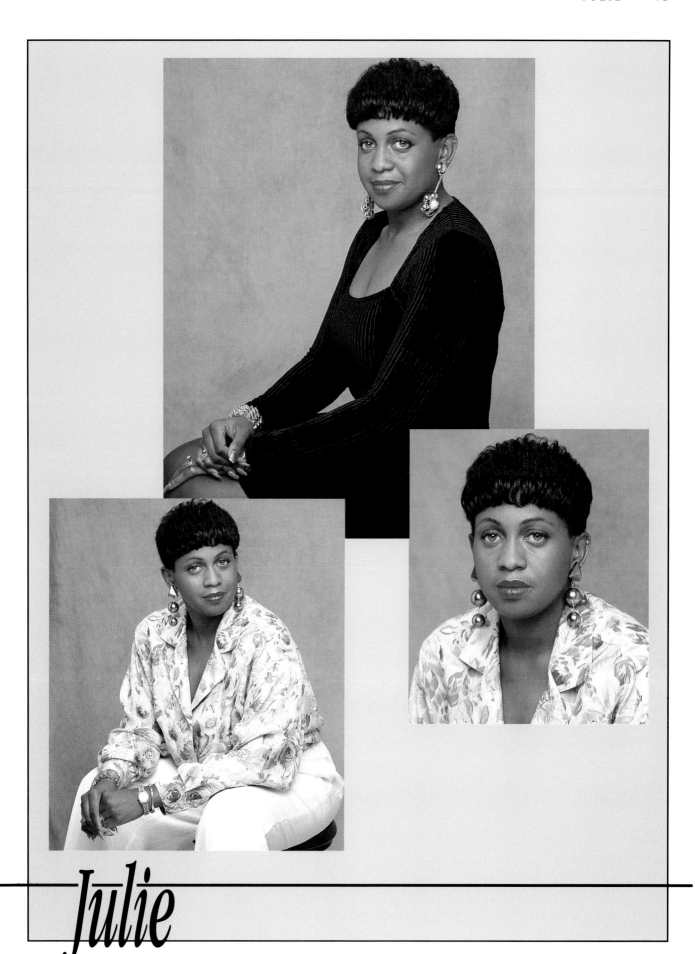

Julie

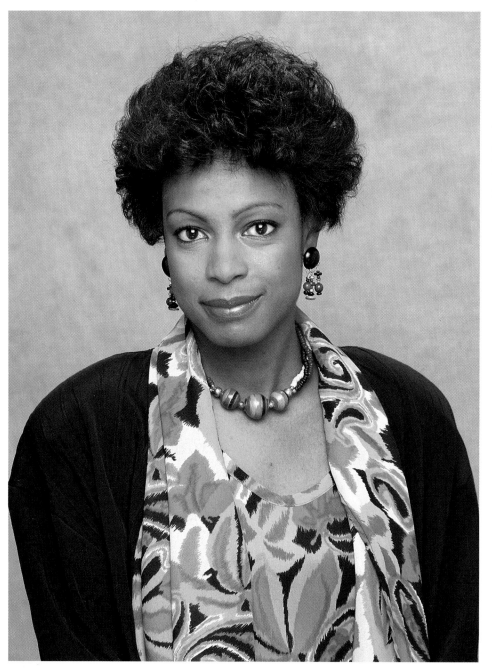

Throughout history the name "Mary" denotes refined charm, grace, and femininity. A hairstyle for such a lady must have the same qualities.

No. *4* *Mary*

SERVICES

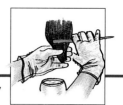

CHEMICAL RELAXER
THERMAL CURLING

TECHNICAL REFERENCE NUMBER 106, 107

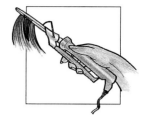

The most sought after hair-care service by women (and men) with excessively curly hair is the "relaxer." Some or most of the tight curl must be removed in order to give the client a modern hair-style.

Natural Black hair can be straightened or temporarily reformed by using thermal irons of various types, but the hair reverts to its natural state when it is exposed to moisture.

Relaxer products are refined to a point of extreme safety and effectiveness when applied by a skilled technician. Black women have a wide variety of fashionable styles from which to choose.

One of the most important factors in a successful relaxer service is the selection of the product. That will be determined by a skilled analysis of the hair and scalp.

Mary's personal hair analysis is permanently recorded.

MARY											
HAIR ANALYSIS											
Natural Texture: Wave ☐ Curl ☑ Kink ☐											
Previous Chemical Service: Relaxed ☑ Straightened ☐ Colored ☐											
Code:	1	2	3	4	5	6	7	8	9	10	
Porosity						✓					
Elasticity						✓					
Density				✓							
Coarseness					✓						
Hair Condition			✓								
Scalp Condition	✓										
Existing Gray	○										
Technical Reference Number	**106**			**107**							
Code based on a scale number 1–10 #1 = Good/Average #10 = Poor/Abnormal											

SERVICE RECOMMENDED

RELAXER TOUCH-UP

Used to decrease the amount of curl at the scalp and utilize the existing hair length to best style advantage.

PROCEDURE

Based on the analysis a mild, no-base relaxer is selected. Protective cream is applied to the skin around the hairline, taking care not to rub it onto the hair. The out-growth is only one-half inch. Extreme care must be taken not to overlap that length and accidentally apply relaxer to previously relaxed hair — the principle cause of breakage.

1 Divide the hair into four or more, easy-to-handle sections. Outline only the back sections. Apply relaxer as near the scalp as possible without actually touching the scalp.

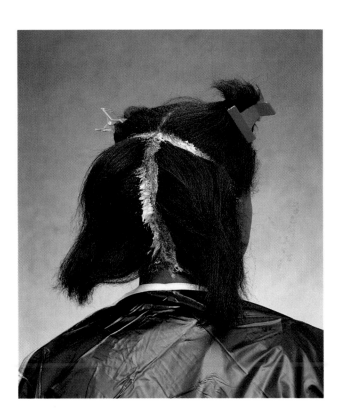

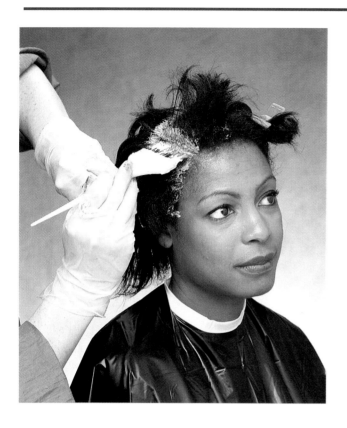

2 Use an applicator brush for fast, even distribution. Start at the top of one of the back sections and make narrow horizontal parts. Apply relaxer only to the new growth, making sure you can see the relaxer through the narrow panel.

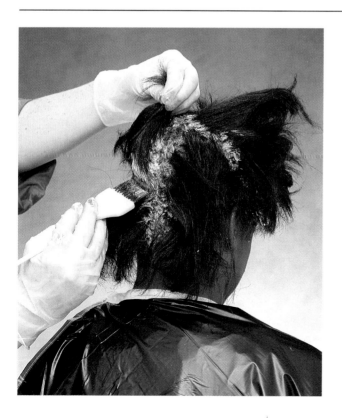

3 When relaxer has been applied to both back sections, move to the front and repeat the application procedure.

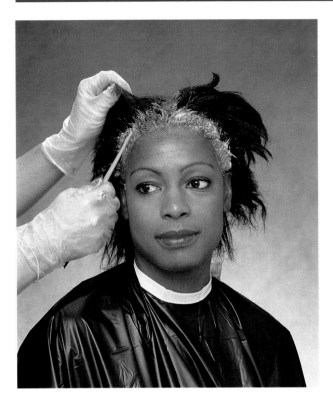

4 Once the relaxer application is completed, go back over each panel, applying tension to the hair with the back of the comb and a gloved finger.

Note: When the hair appears to be straight or slightly wavy when smoothed, immediately rinse all product from the hair with warm, not hot, water. Follow with a gentle neutralizing shampoo and conditioner. The hair is now ready for styling.

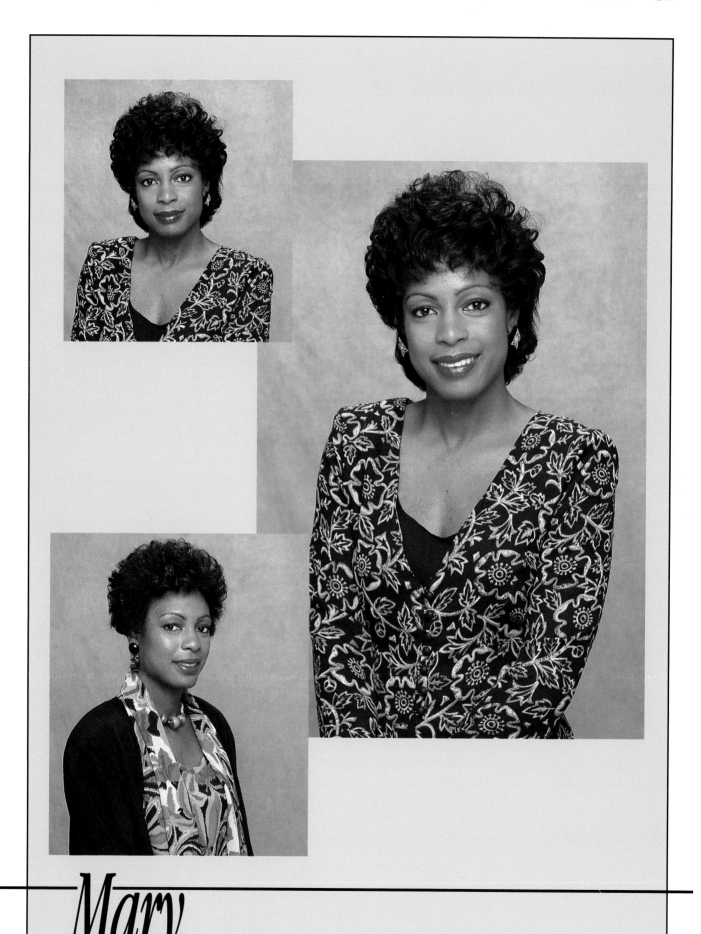

Mary

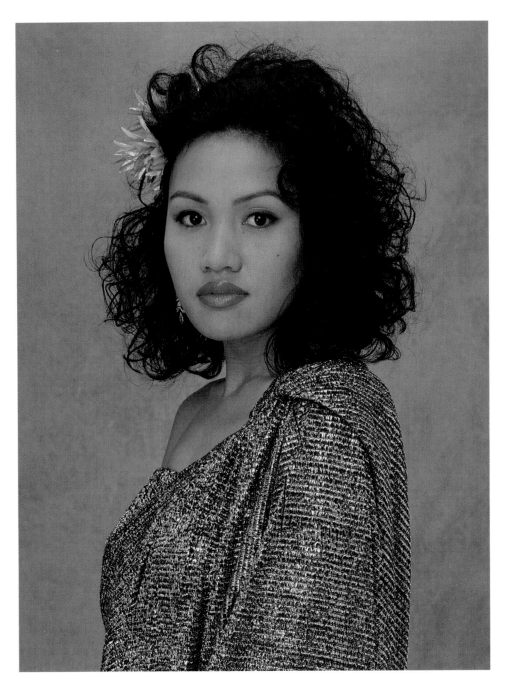

Hair is the focus of feminine beauty. Celebrate the spirit of youth and romance at every opportunity.

No. 5 *Vichett*

SERVICES

PERM/CURL RE-FORMATION

TECHNICAL REFERENCE NUMBER 106

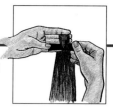

Vichett's virgin hair has uniform waves about one-half inch wide throughout. The hair is sufficiently fine and pliable that a standard perm using a large diameter perm rod will sufficiently extend the curl formation to approximately an inch wide. This will allow the hair to be dried naturally or styled in a variety of ways not possible with such narrow wave pattern.

It is not unusual that hair of Black women is not kinky or matted at the scalp. Instead the hair closely resembles that of a Caucasian having excessive curl. That type hair can easily be re-formed using a thio perm solution formulated for resistant hair.

However, in order to be sure the desired effect was obtained, the technician presoftened the hair at the shampoo bowl prior to perming. She simply foamed thio perm lotion into the hair and used her gloved fingers to stretch the hair somewhat. That procedure removed some of the curl and made the hair more receptive to the actual perm process.

Vichett's hair analysis becomes a permanent record for future hair care services.

VICHETT

HAIR ANALYSIS

Natural Texture: Wave ☑   Curl ☐   Kink ☐

Previous Chemical Service: Relaxed ☑   Straightened ☐   Colored ☐

Code:	1	2	3	4	5	6	7	8	9	10	
Porosity			✓								
Elasticity		✓									
Density					✓						
Coarseness				✓							
Hair Condition		✓									
Scalp Condition	✓										
Existing Gray	○										

Technical Reference Number   **106**

Code based on a scale number 1–10

#1 = Good/Average

#10 = Poor/Abnormal

SERVICE RECOMMENDED

CURL RE-FORMATION USING A STANDARD PERM PROCEDURE

Used to make the narrow natural wave pattern wider to respond to more contemporary styling.

PROCEDURE

Unless the hair has a lot of spray or grease on it, no shampoo is necessary before a perm of this type.

Keeping in mind that the finished circle of the re-formed curl will be approximately one and one-half times the diameter of the rod, make your rod selection on that basis.

1 Divide the hair into panels equally as wide as the perm rod is long. Subsection for rod placement no wider than the diameter of the rod being used. Start wrapping in area of the head with the strongest curl. In this instance the technician chose to start at the back of the hair line at a part slightly off center.

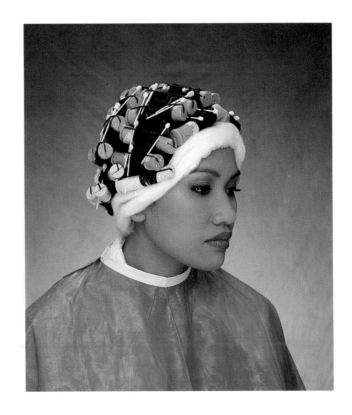

2 Continue wrapping, placing each rod on its own base and applying medium tension from ends to the scalp. Direct the rods from the center down toward the hairline directly in line with the section being wrapped. Continue the procedure until all hair has been wrapped.

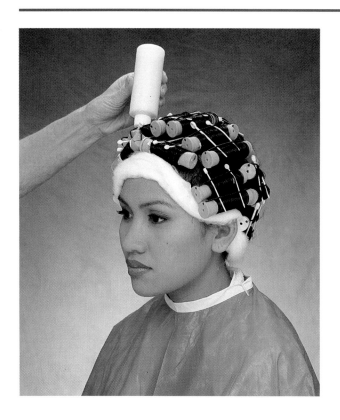

3 Position a protective cotton strip around the hairline to prevent solution from running onto the skin. Thoroughly saturate the hair around each perm rod.

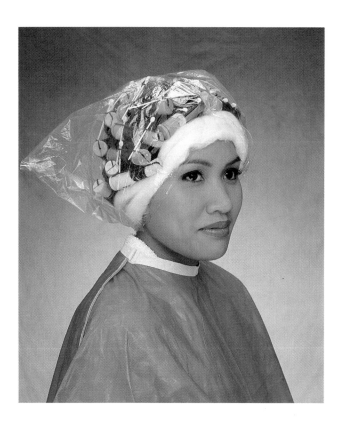

4 Place a plastic processing cap over the rods and process the perm according to manufacturer's instructions. Take frequent test curls in different areas of the head to test curl development.

Note: When the perm has processed to its full potential, neutralize as instructed, lightly shampoo and condition the hair, and it is ready for styling.

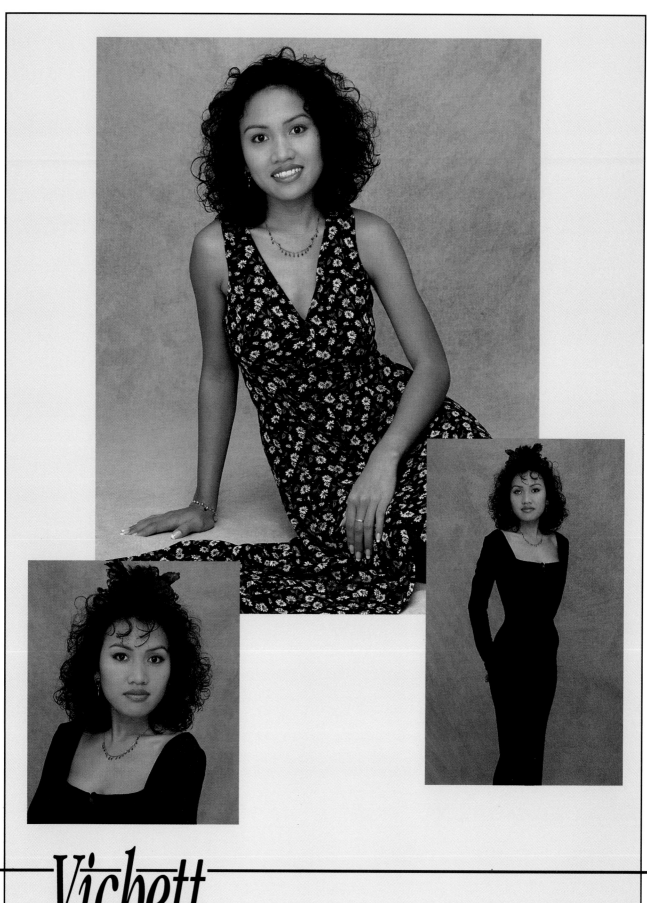

Vichett

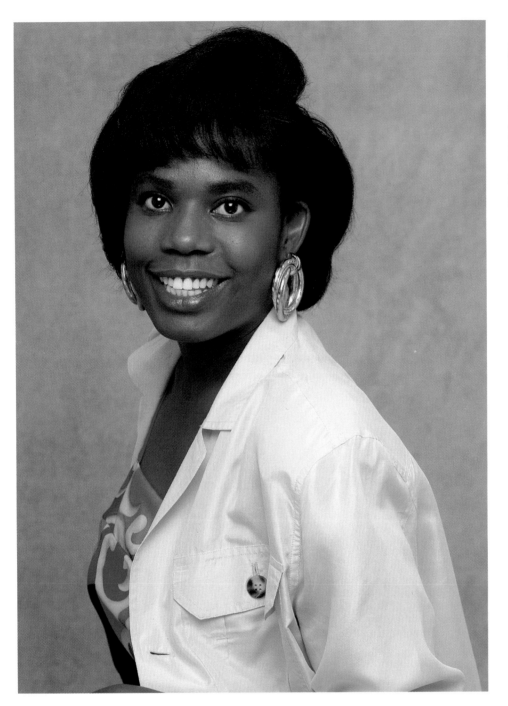

O ne's hairstyle should reflect or even encourage a latent personality trait. A happy, playful person needs to feel as well as look the part.

No. *6* *Tammie*

SERVICES

THERMAL STYLING
IRON-CURLING

TECHNICAL REFERENCE NUMBER 107

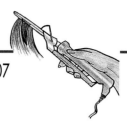

Tammie's hair has been chemically relaxed. Her weekly hair care service most often includes a deep cleansing shampoo and conditioner, after which the hair is carefully blown dry and iron curled.

Hot comb and pressing (thermal styling) is the oldest salon service for temporarily straightening Black hair. However, hot irons in inexperienced hands can cause a lot of damage including singed hair, breakage, and scalp burns.

Most thermal iron mistakes are due to lack of knowledge regarding the implements used. Never apply heat to hair without first testing the appliance. Hair can withstand heat only to a certain tempera-

ture without burning. Irons heated to 380 to 400 degrees are too hot for most hair types. It is important to cool the irons before using.

Another important factor in judging the correct temperature of thermal irons to be used on an individual's hair is the personal hair analysis. Fine textured hair needs much less heat than medium or thick textured manes. Never make the mistake of assuming all Black hair is the same. The texture, density, elasticity, and porosity vary considerably.

Tammie's personal hair analysis is permanently recorded.

TAMMIE											
HAIR ANALYSIS											
Natural Texture: Wave ☐ Curl ☐ Kink ☑											
Previous Chemical Service: Relaxed ☑ Straightened ☐ Colored ☐											
Code:	1	2	3	4	5	6	7	8	9	10	
Porosity					✓						
Elasticity					✓						
Density					✓						
Coarseness							✓				
Hair Condition			✓								
Scalp Condition	✓										
Existing Gray	○										
Technical Reference Number	**107**										

Code based on a scale number 1–10
#1 = Good/Average
#10 = Poor/Abnormal

SERVICE RECOMMENDED

STYLE CONSTRUCTION BY THERMAL IRON METHOD

A quick, easy way to create a contemporary hairstyle in relaxed, medium short hair.

PROCEDURE

Note: The barrel size of the iron is selected according to the length of hair and the desired result. For a smooth hairstyle with minimum curl, a large diameter iron was used.

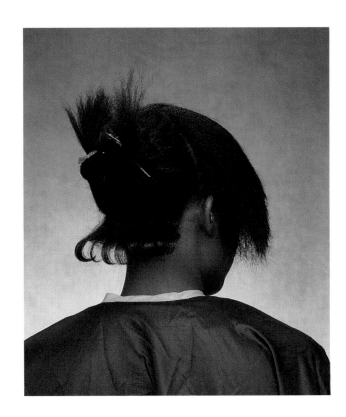

1 After cleansing, conditioning, and blowing the hair dry, divide into easy to handle sections. For rapid iron curling, sections no wider than the length of the barrel of the iron are preferred by most stylists.

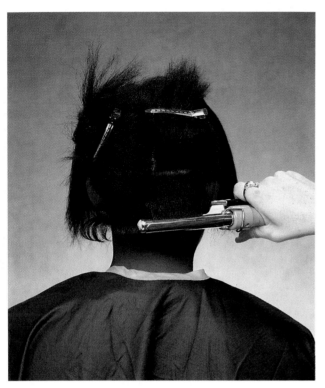

2 Turn the hair at the nape under. Slide the half open iron down the hair strand and make only a half turn on the ends.

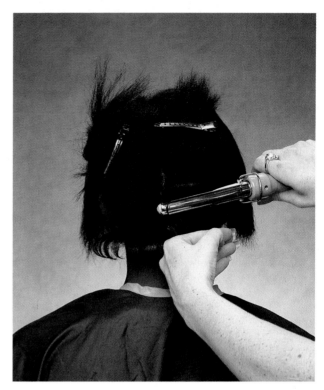

3 The same basic design principles apply for making "heat" curls as for positioning rollers for a wet set. An on-base curl creates volume and decreases with the degree of lift.

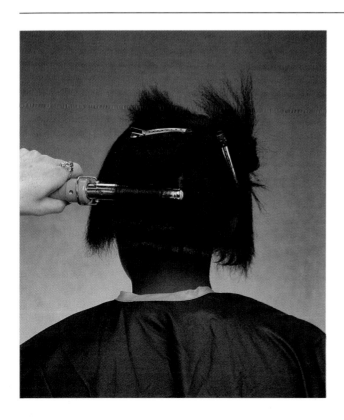

4 Hold the hair at approximately forty-five degrees from the head for curling the hair from the nape to the lower crown.

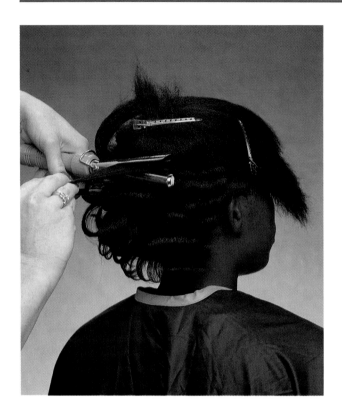

5 Alternate from side to side and roll all the hair in the back, gradually increasing the volume in the crown area.

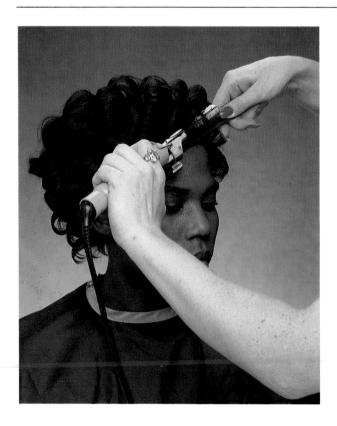

6 Curl the hair on top, in front, and on the sides from the crown toward the corresponding hairline.

Note: When the iron curls have all been formed allow the hair to cool completely before brushing and combing into style.

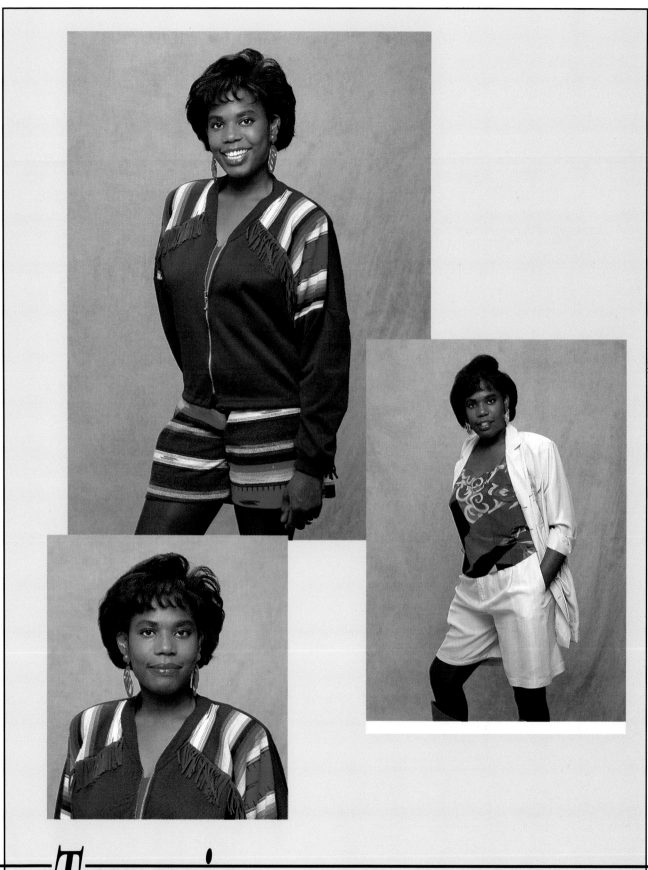

Tammie

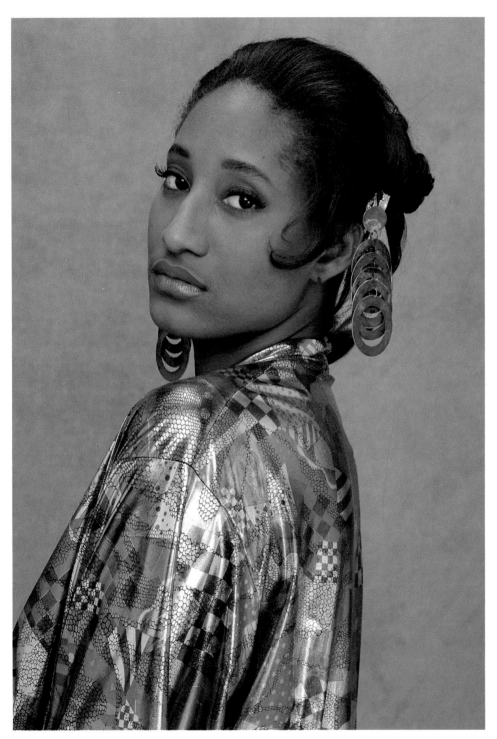

A dramatic, intricately ornamented hairstyle often inhibits a naturally shy person. Carefully select a confident person — one, perhaps, whose name is Diedra.

No. 7 *Diedra*

SERVICES

FLAT PRESSING
HAIR EXTENSION

TECHNICAL REFERENCE NUMBER 108, 110

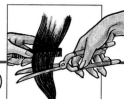

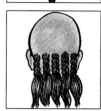

Diedra's natural hair is short due to breakage resulting from an over-processed relaxer and a high-lift color treatment.

Because she looks and feels better in long hair, she opts for an abundance of faux hair while her own grows to an adaptable length.

The hair used to extend the length of Diedra's shortened locks is made of synthetic fiber that looks much like real human hair. There are definite advantages to synthetic wefts. Human hair is considerably more expensive than synthetic fiber. The care of synthetic extensions is simple because it is lightweight and easily cleansed with mild detergent. It needs no conditioning. Real human hair requires the same conditioning on a regular basis as hair growing on the head.

There's also at least one disadvantage to the use of synthetic extensions — they do not respond to standard methods of styling. They can, however, be smoothed somewhat with a flat pressing iron kept at a very moderate temperature.

As a professional it is your duty to give the best service possible to each and every client — under good and not-so-good conditions. Diedra's problem is real and you will have a steadfast, loyal client if you will keep her looking as good as possible while her own hair grows.

Diedra's hair analysis becomes a permanent record as a guide for future hair care services.

DIEDRA

HAIR ANALYSIS

Natural Texture: Wave ☐   Curl ☐   Kink ☑

Previous Chemical Service: Relaxed ☐   Straightened ☑   Colored ☑

Code:	1	2	3	4	5	6	7	8	9	10	
Porosity						✓					
Elasticity							✓				
Density							✓				
Coarseness								✓			
Hair Condition						✓					
Scalp Condition	✓										
Existing Gray	○										
Technical Reference Number		**108**			**110**						

Code based on a scale number 1–10

#1 = Good/Average

#10 = Poor/Abnormal

SERVICE RECOMMENDED

**SECURING PREVIOUSLY ATTACHED WEFTS
AND FLAT PRESSING THE EXTENDED SYNTHETIC
HAIR INTO A STYLE AS SMOOTH AS POSSIBLE**

Done to create the appearance of a full, natural hair growth.

PROCEDURE

Note: Preheat the pressing iron while you retie the wefts where needed. Use a pressing iron that has a thermostat setting. Heat the iron only to a low temperature not to exceed 100 degrees Fahrenheit. If the iron is too hot it will singe (burn) the synthetic fabric wherever it is touched by the iron.

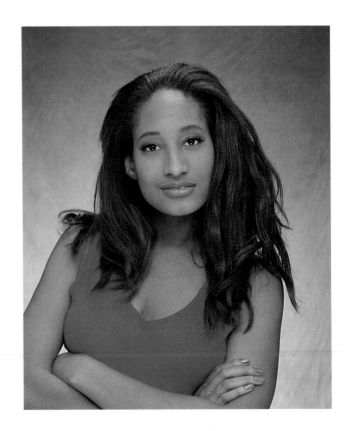

1 Before. The hair wefts used for extended length need to be brushed, combed, and pressed smooth to look their best.

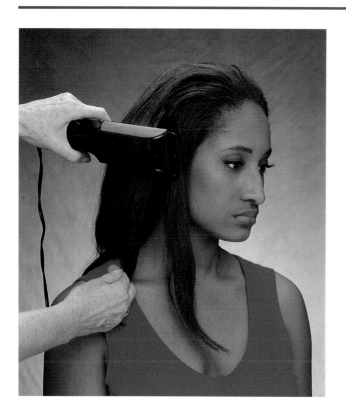

2 Use your little finger to pull out a narrow panel of hair for pressing. Insert the OPEN iron where the natural hair ends and the weft nearest the crown begins. Close the iron as it moves down the strand. Never hold the iron in one place — keep it moving at all times.

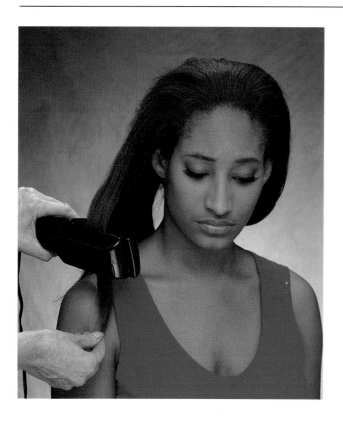

3 Continue to pull the closed iron down toward the ends of the hair. Curve the iron slightly toward the head so the hair will have a tendency to turn under.

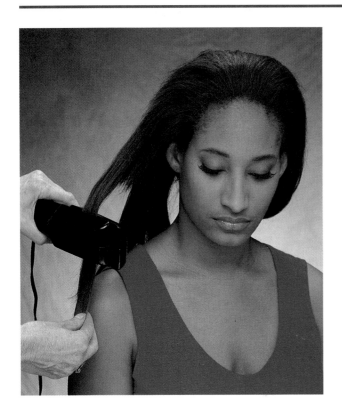

4 Hold the hair away from the client as you move the iron as a precaution against burning her neck or shoulder. Repeat the pressing procedure until all the hair has been smoothed. Go over previously pressed strands if necessary to get the desired effect.

Note: Don't expect miracles. As we discussed, synthetic hair does not respond as well as real human hair. If the client wants perfectly straight extended length, be sure to order the wefts in that condition. They will need attention once they are attached.

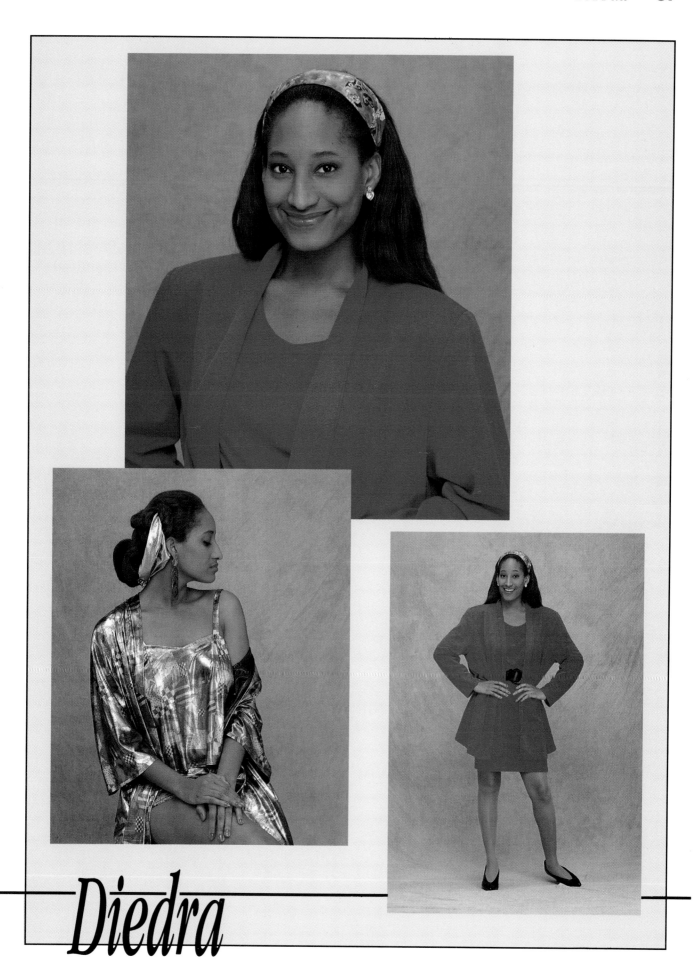

Diedra

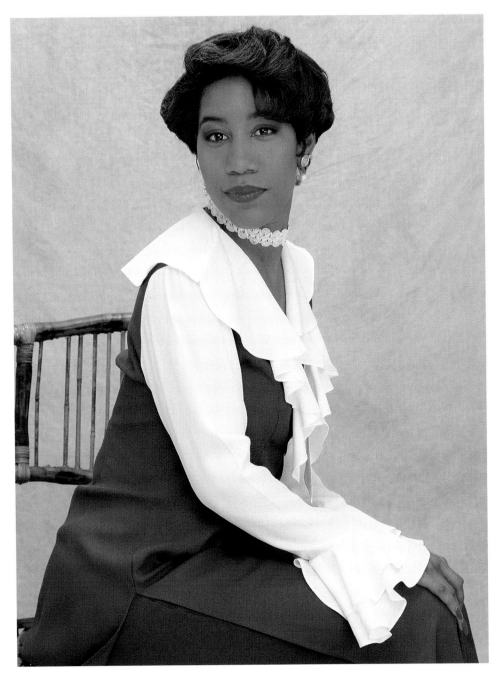

Fashion awareness is the mark of many modern career women who will settle for nothing less than current hairstyles quickly executed and easily maintained.

Christine

SERVICES

QUICK PRESS
PRESSING COMB

TECHNICAL REFERENCE NUMBER 109

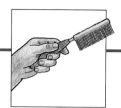

Black hair that has only medium-tight curl and a fine texture is a prime candidate for most quick-service techniques.

Pressing is only one method of attaining a smooth surface while creating lift and volume in specific areas of a hairstyle. A professional technician, having the ability to skillfully manipulate a pressing comb, can create rounded curl formations resembling those made with a curling iron.

Prior to this pressing service, Christine's hair was chemically relaxed. The hair was conditioned and cut into an attractive style having a fitted nape and a strategically placed weight line. Pressing is simply a way of quickly servicing this client's hair care needs between major chemical treatments. She is an ideal client who shows off a stylist's work to the very best advantage.

Christine's personal hair and scalp analysis will become a permanent record for future services. Even though you have an individual's analysis record on file, you must carefully examine the hair and scalp each time she visits the salon. A careful examination will detect any changes that should be noted before giving a specific service.

CHRISTINE

HAIR ANALYSIS

Natural Texture: Wave ☐   Curl ☑   Kink ☐

Previous Chemical Service: Relaxed ☐   Straightened ☑   Colored ☑

Code:	1	2	3	4	5	6	7	8	9	10	
Porosity			✓								
Elasticity					✓						
Density					✓						
Coarseness		✓									
Hair Condition		✓									
Scalp Condition	✓										
Existing Gray	○										
Technical Reference Number	**109**										

Code based on a scale number 1–10

#1 = Good/Average

#10 = Poor/Abnormal

SERVICE RECOMMENDED

A "QUICK-PRESS"

Done to emphasize the form, smooth the surface, and create an attractive hairstyle.

PROCEDURE

Note: Be sure the pressing comb is clean and free of residue from styling lotions. Select an electric pressing comb that has a thermostat. Preheat the comb to medium hot. Test the temperature carefully before applying it to the hair. Wrap a white piece of paper tightly around the rounded edge of the comb. If it scorches the paper, the comb is too hot. Allow the comb to cool and turn the temperature control to a lower setting.

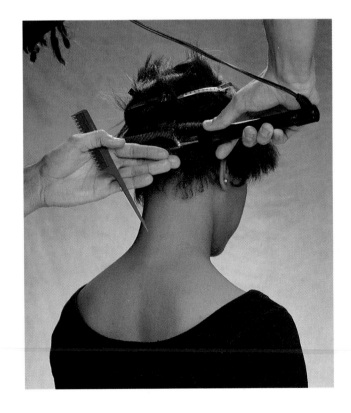

1 Clip the upper portion of the hair out of the way and insert the pressing comb — teeth up — into the hair at the nape area.

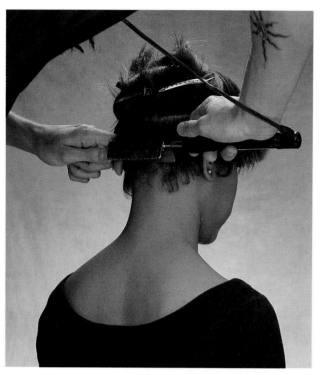

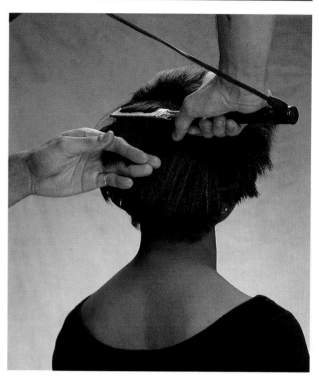

2 As you pull the comb through the strand of hair from the scalp toward the end, turn the teeth of the comb forward until the rounded back of the comb presses against the hair strand. It is the back (the barrel) of the comb that presses the hair — not the teeth.

3 Continue the same pressing procedure up the back of the head. As you work up toward the crown, hold the hair up from the head and slightly overdirect the base to create volume.

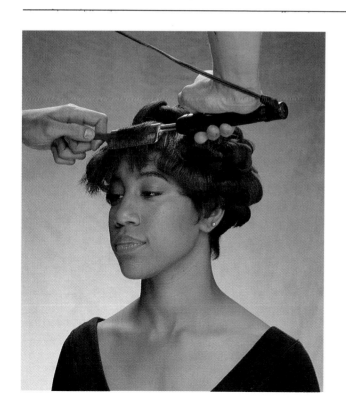

4 Work up each side and into the crown. Each strand that is pressed should result in a complete circle toward the ends of the hair. This is accomplished by turning the comb down and in a circle toward the head to create a soft curl formation.

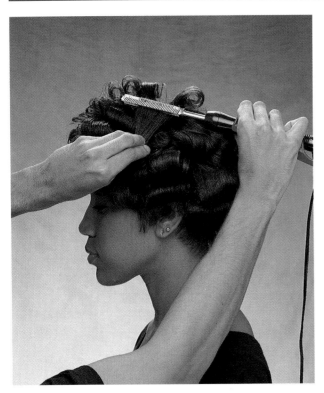

5 The front area is the last to be pressed. Complete the pressing procedure by the same method used throughout.

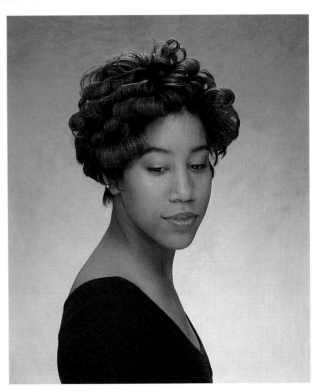

6 In viewing the completed press, examine the hair throughout to any area, especially around the perimeter, that may need an additional touch-up.

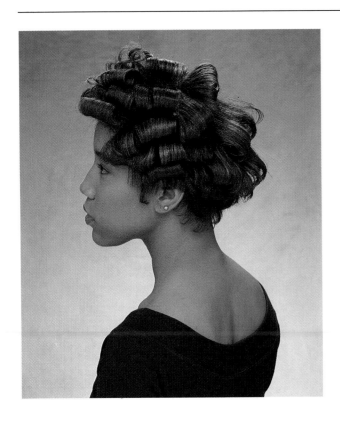

7 Be sure the hair is thoroughly cooled before brushing and combing it into style.

FINISHED STYLES:

This particular haircut may be styled in a variety of ways that is flattering to the client.

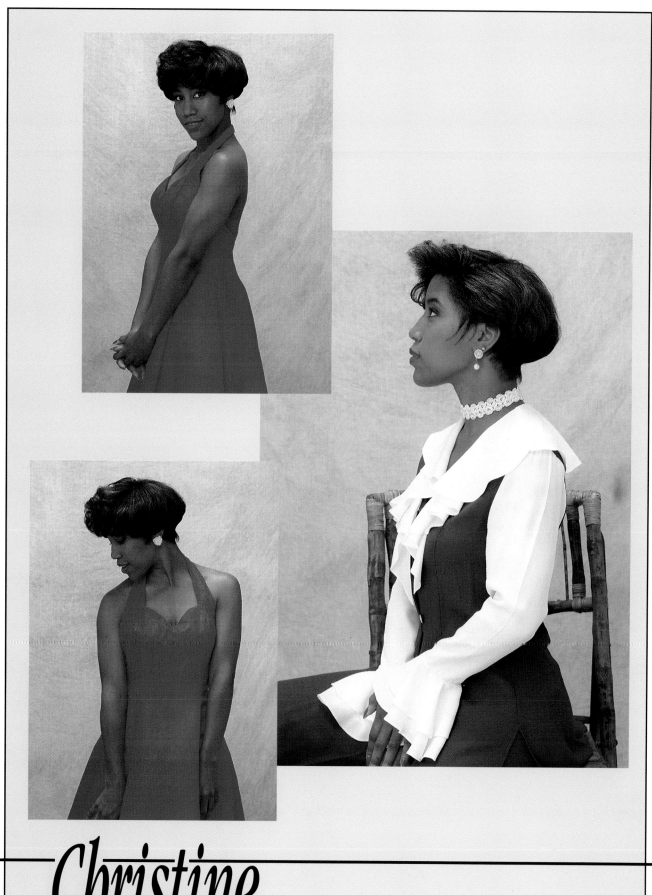

Christine

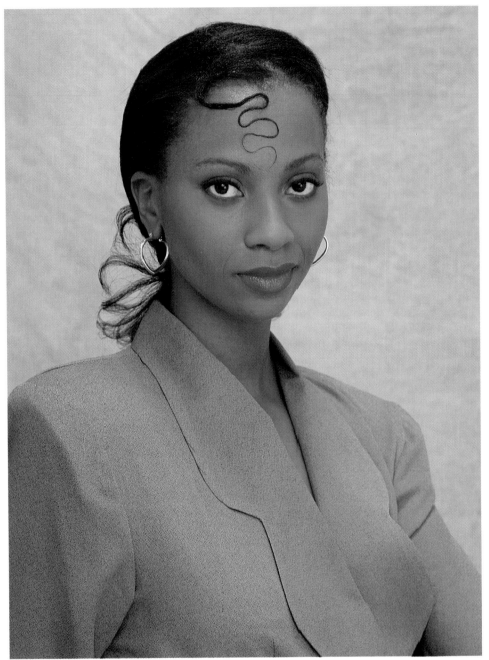

C hic, sophisticated hairstyles, with a focus that distinctly sets them apart, are favored by women climbing the ladder of success.

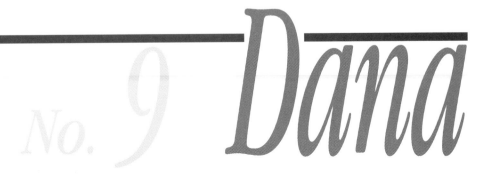

No. 9 *Dana*

SERVICES

SHAMPOO
CONDITIONER
BLOW DRY
THERMAL FINISH

TECHNICAL REFERENCE NUMBER 101, 102, 104, 107

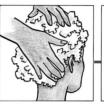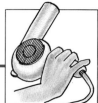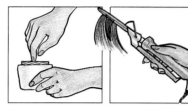

Even hair that has been chemically straightened will not have a smooth surface unless it is air-formed or heat processed after a shampoo.

To wear a smooth-surface hairstyle, Dana's hair is first shampooed, conditioned, and then blown dry until it is straight, smooth, and shiny.

Blow drying curly hair while applying tension with a round styling brush temporarily re-forms the hair structure. Physical bonds in the hair are broken by the water used for shampooing. While the hair is wet (damp) it can be stretched and dried using this heat source. However, the straight effect is temporary. When the hair is wet again the curl will return.

Dana's personal hair analysis determines the service required and the limitations and care that must be taken during such service. This analysis should become a permanent record for future services to this client.

DANA

HAIR ANALYSIS

Natural Texture: Wave ☐   Curl ☐   Kink ☑

Previous Chemical Service: Relaxed ☐   Straightened ☑   Colored ☐

Code:	1	2	3	4	5	6	7	8	9	10	
Porosity							✓				
Elasticity							✓				
Density						✓					
Coarseness					✓						
Hair Condition					✓						
Scalp Condition	✓										
Existing Gray	○										

| Technical Reference Number | **101** | **102** | **104** | **107** |

Code based on a scale number 1–10
#1 = Good/Average
#10 = Poor/Abnormal

SERVICE RECOMMENDED

Due to excellent hair condition, any preferred technique used to create a current hairstyle is safe and appropriate. Air forming is considered the most effective method for the client's style request.

PROCEDURE

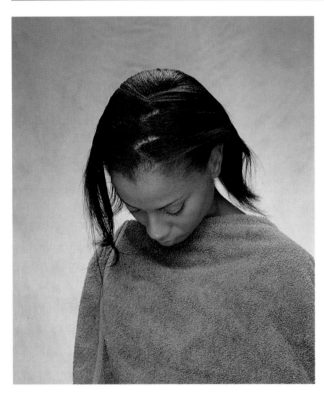

Because the hair has been chemically straightened, there's no need to twist and apply pressure at the scalp to remove excess curl. The blow drying procedure will dry, smooth, and direct the hair sufficiently for styling.

1 Divide the hair by making a zig-zag center part. This encourages the hair to fall naturally over the curves of the head as it is blown dry.

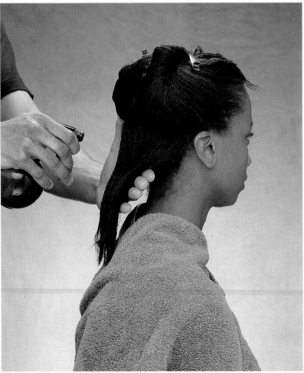

2 Make a horizontal part from ear to ear just above the occipital bone. Spray lightly with thermal styling lotion.

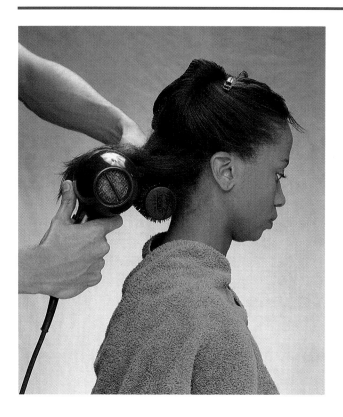

3 Use the hand-held dryer to pick up a section of hair from underneath the strand. Hold the hair while positioning the round brush.

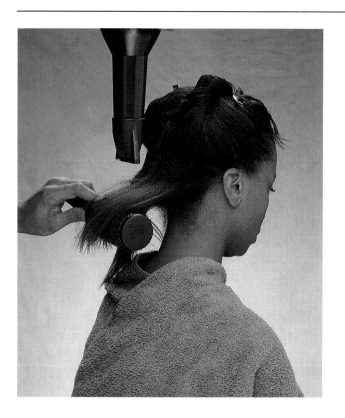

4 Start turning the brush under as it is pulled through the hair from scalp to hair ends. Hold the blow dryer a few inches away from the hair, direct the air flow onto the hair being held, and follow the brush down the strand. (Turn the temperature control to medium to guard against burning the hair.)

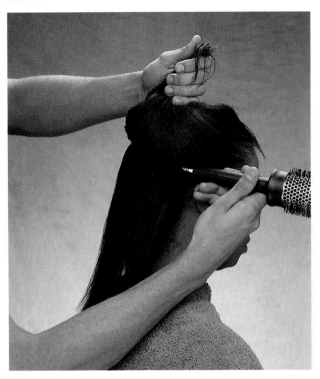

5 When the nape section is thoroughly dried, part off a second horizontal section. Let down a narrow panel of hair and blow it dry using the same procedure.

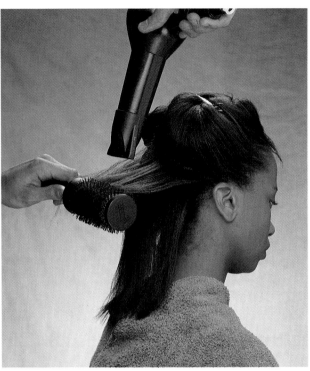

6 Be sure each strand of hair is thoroughly dry, straight, and silky smooth before proceeding to another section.

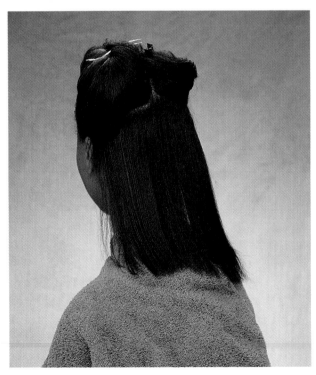

7 When the back has been blown dry, part the crown into easy-to-handle sections.

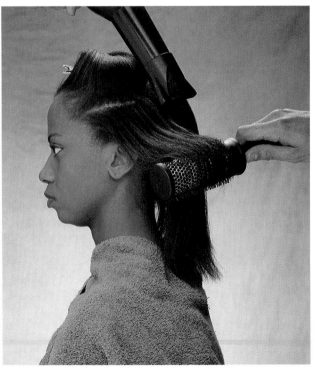

8 Work from side to side letting down narrow panels of hair and blowing each into style line.

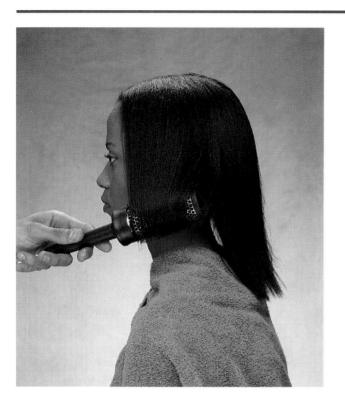

9 Finish blow drying by smoothing the sides and the frontal areas. Apply a small amount of hairdressing creme and go back over the entire surface for added smoothness and shine.

IRON CURL FINISH

Note: The object is to turn the ends slightly up as for a flip.

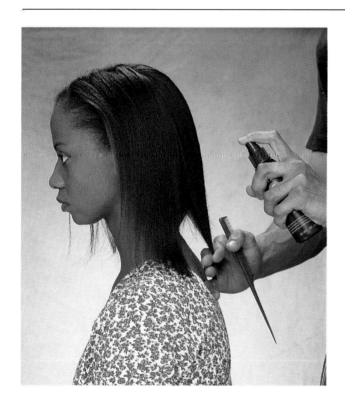

10 Spray the ends lightly with heat protection lotion.

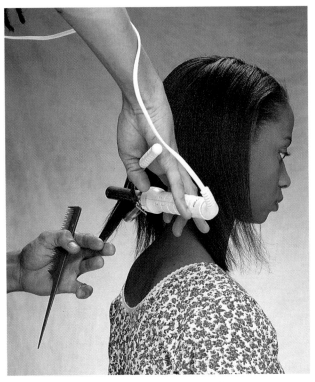

11 Insert the large barrel curling iron into a section of hair in the center back. Be sure the groove of the iron is on the bottom. Keep the irons open slightly and pull them down the strand toward the ends

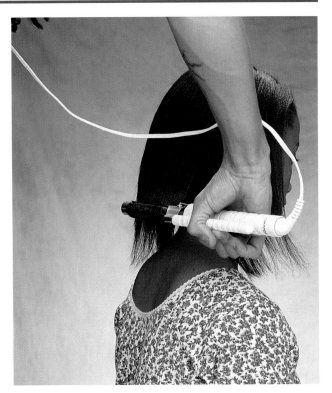

12 Turn the irons up, one half turn, to make sure the ends are caught smoothly between the groove and the barrel. Make one more complete turn and hold for a few seconds. Feel the hair over the iron with your fingers to avoid excess heat.

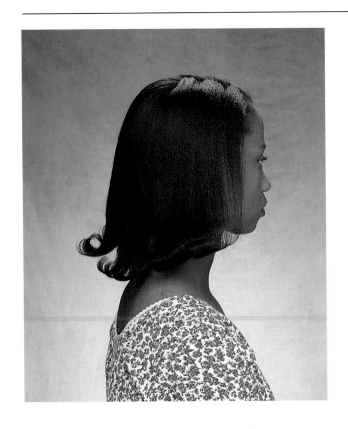

13 Continue all around the perimeter of the otherwise straight hair until the ends have been turned slightly up.

Note: Let the hair cool completely and brush and/or comb it into the desired style. Because the hair is in a natural fall, it can easily be styled in a variety of ways.

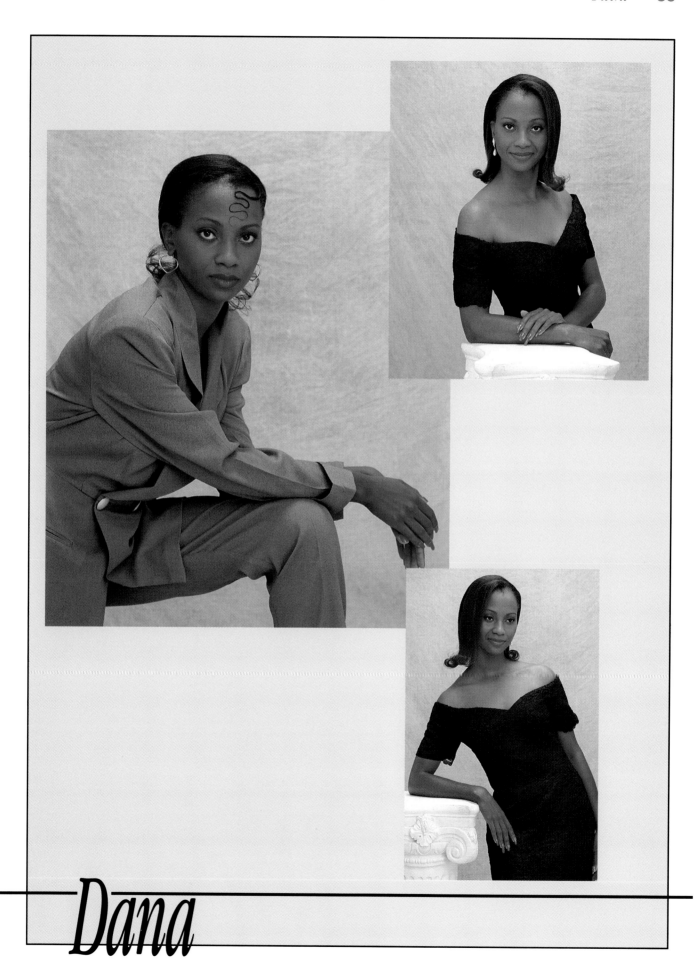

Dana

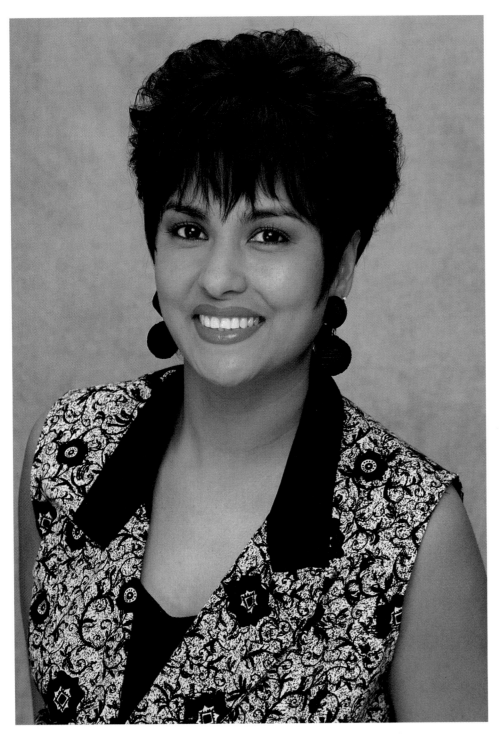

A quintessential classic look is perennially favored by women who want to make a smart but subtle fashion statement.

No. 10 *Riaana*

SERVICES

RELAXER/PERM

TECHNICAL REFERENCE NUMBER 106

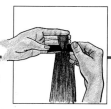

Some hair types simply do not respond well to "hot" design tools. Riaana's hair is extremely fine, having only medium density and a medium amount of curl. Most of the curl is in the crown area.

For all those reasons the existing curl is removed by using an ammonium thioglycolic relaxer as opposed to the more abrasive sodium hydroxide variety.

By using a "thio" product to remove excess curl, the hair can then be re-formed by means of a standard perm-rod technique, thus creating volume without curl.

When servicing a Black clientele it is well to remember that not all Black women (or men) are of African decent. Many have a background of mixed ethnic heritage. This accounts for different hair textures and skin tones. As a professional, you will know by examining the hair and scalp the strength of the chemical to use for the desired effect.

Riaana's personal hair analysis becomes a permanent record for all future hair care services.

RIAANA

HAIR ANALYSIS

Natural Texture: Wave ☑   Curl ☐   Kink ☐

Previous Chemical Service: Relaxed ☑   Straightened ☐   Colored ☐

Code:	1	2	3	4	5	6	7	8	9	10	
Porosity			✓								
Elasticity			✓								
Density					✓						
Coarseness		✓									
Hair Condition	✓										
Scalp Condition	✓										
Existing Gray	○										

Technical Reference Number	**106**			

Code based on a scale number 1–10

#1 = Good/Average

#10 = Poor/Abnormal

SERVICES RECOMMENDED

**A MILD THIOGLYCOLIC RELAXER
FOLLOWED BY
A THIO PERM USING LARGE ROLLERS**

The relaxer is used to remove unwanted curl and create straight lines at the perimeter and volume in the crown.

PROCEDURE

Note: The hair should be free from excess oils, finishing lotions, and sprays before a mild "thio" relaxer is used. If it is necessary to shampoo the hair, be very careful not to rub the scalp. Squeeze the shampoo through the hair only and rinse thoroughly with slightly warm water. Towel dry to remove excess moisture.

RELAXER

NOT SHOWN:
Apply relaxer by using a standard application technique. Comb through the hair using your gloved hand as well, until the hair appears perfectly straight around the perimeter and only a slight wave remains in the crown area.

When the hair is sufficiently relaxed once again, carefully remove all chemical product from the hair and towel blot all excess moisture, leaving the hair only slightly damp.

CURL REFORMATION

The same strength perm solution may be used to restructure the curl formation as used as a relaxer. Select rollers having a diameter that allows the hair to go around two complete turns. Use plastic-coated clips to secure the rods, and use two or more end papers to wrap each curl. The paper keeps the hair secure and provides a degree of tension.

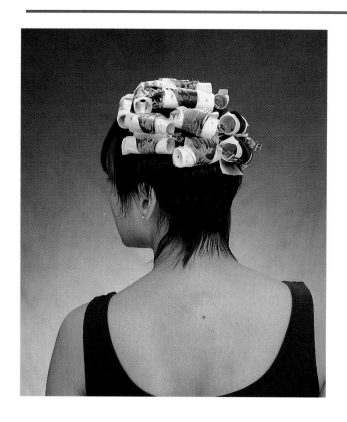

1 Comb all the perimeter hair flat and straight. Block off a circular area including the crown and the natural curve of the head. Using two end papers for each rod, start wrapping from a center point just behind the bangs.

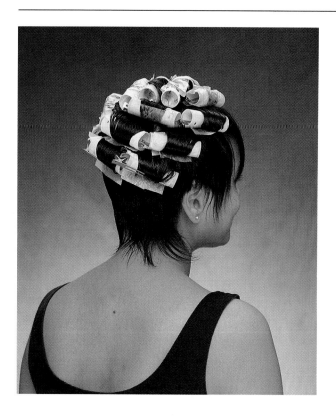

2 Continue to direct each rod slightly down and toward the back to conform to the natural head form.

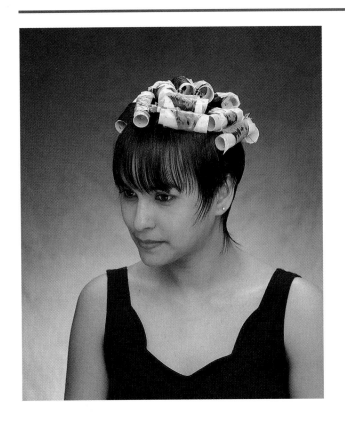

3 Place all rods in center crown directly on base, keeping as much tension as possible with oversized rods.

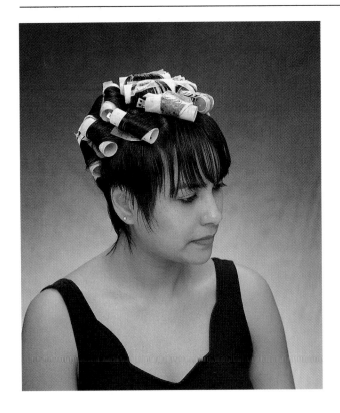

4 Follow the natural head form and perm down to and including the occipital bone area. All perimeter hair is left hanging straight.

Note: Process the perm according to manufacturer's instructions. When the process is complete, shampoo the hair lightly and spray with conditioning styling lotion. Use a wide bristle vent brush, a cool air dryer, and your fingers to create a lovely hairstyle that can easily be worn on or off the face.

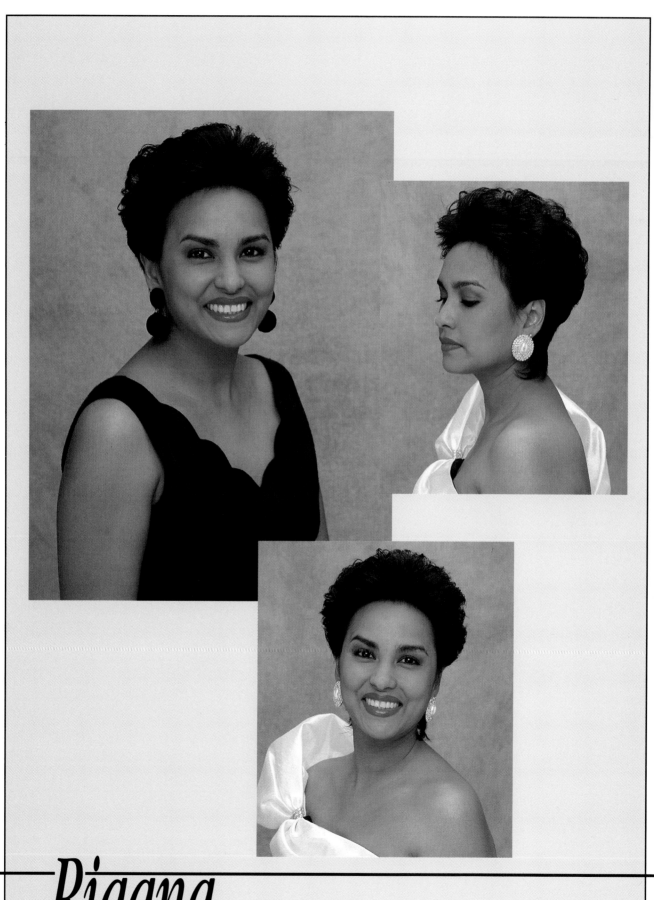

Riaana

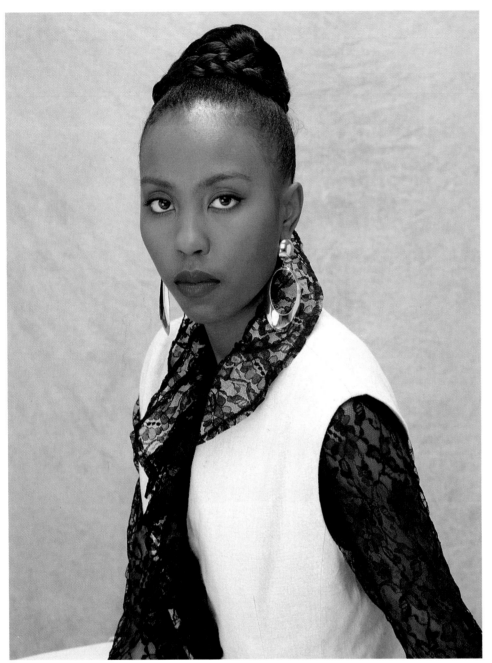

A simple, uncompli- cated hairstyle that can be con- verted to dramatic, understated elegance for special occasions is pre- ferred by many on-the-go career women.

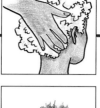
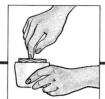
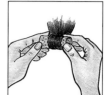
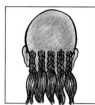

SERVICES

SHAMPOO TECHNICAL REFERENCE NUMBER 101, 102, 103, 110
CONDITIONER
STYLE
EXTENSION

Theresa is a professional model whose livelihood depends, quite literally, on her physical appearance. She places a great value on her hairdresser, whom she counts on to keep her hair in excellent condition and simply, but smartly styled.

Black hair that must be chemically relaxed is quite limited when it comes to hairstyles that require minimum maintenance. Quite simply, very kinky hair, even after being straightened, will not stay smooth and support a design line without daily care.

The few ways available to Black clients are styles that can be slicked close to the head and held with holding gels and sprays — or one or more of the popular braided styles.

Because Theresa is required by clients who engage her modeling services to look many different ways, she prefers to keep her hair short and add hairpieces such as chignons, ornamental braids, hanging wefts, or swatches or, if necessary, full wigs.

She is a regular client and has several hair care services at different intervals, always scheduled on the advice of her hairdresser.

Her personal hair analysis chart is reviewed before each and every service. Her entire hair history, including dates of individual services, is carefully recorded.

THERESA

HAIR ANALYSIS

Natural Texture: Wave ☐   Curl ☐   Kink ☑

Previous Chemical Service: Relaxed ☑   Straightened ☐   Colored ☐

Code:	1	2	3	4	5	6	7	8	9	10	
Porosity								✓			
Elasticity								✓			
Density						✓					
Coarseness						✓					
Hair Condition					✓						
Scalp Condition	✓										
Existing Gray	○										
Technical Reference Number	**101**			**102**			**103**			**110**	

	Code based on a scale number 1–10	
	#1 = Good/Average	
	#10 = Poor/Abnormal	

SERVICE RECOMMENDED

A deep cleansing shampoo/protein conditioner, followed by a simple but elegant style with added chignon. The hair was chemically relaxed on her last weekly visit.

PROCEDURE

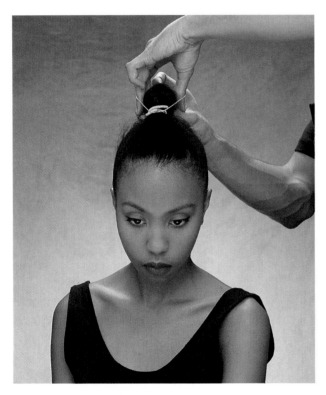

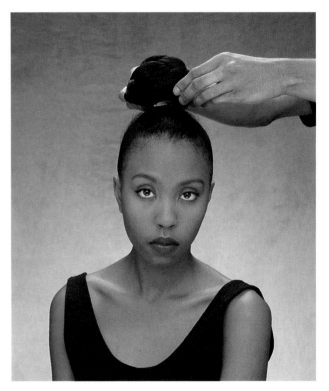

1 The hair is shampooed, blown dry, pulled away from the face, and held with a coated elastic band at the top of the head. When the focus is on curls or chignons at the top of the head, it should be placed at a forty-five degree angle from the chin to the crown for aesthetic balance.

2 A prestyled chignon is placed directly over the hair held at the top.

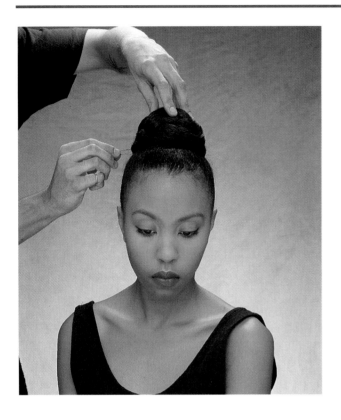

3 Secure the chignon by weaving long hairpins around the edge. Slide the hairpin first through the chignon (about one-half inch from the edge), then into the natural hair. Be careful not to scratch the head while placing the pins.

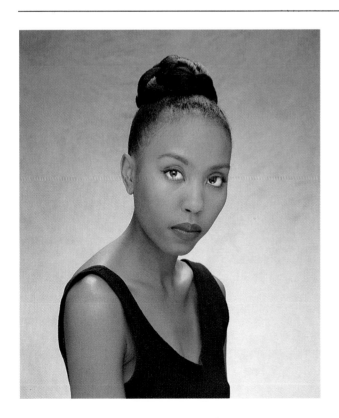

4 Carefully look at the positioned chignon from a front view to be sure it is at the exact angle to flatter the client's features.

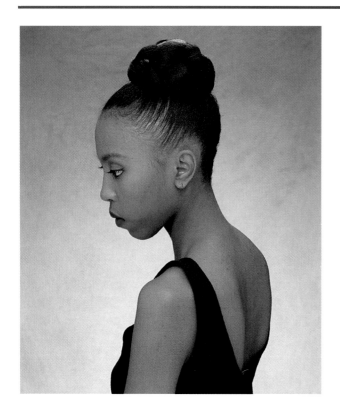

5 Finally, view the placement from a profile. Carefully examine the style to be sure no hairpins are visible.

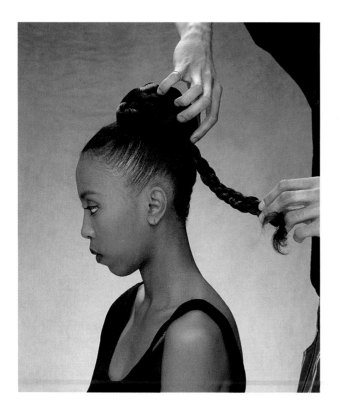

6 The length and diameter of an ornamental braid determines the placement. If the braid is long enough, start by fastening one end of the braid in the center back as close to the chignon as possible.

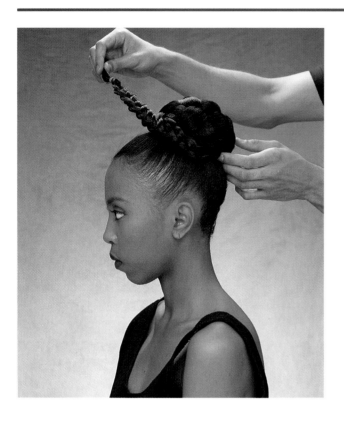

7 Continue to wrap the braid completely around the chignon.

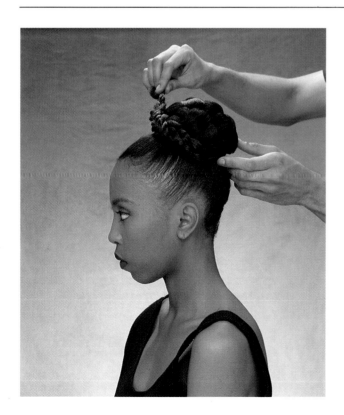

8 Make a second circle with the braid if the length permits.

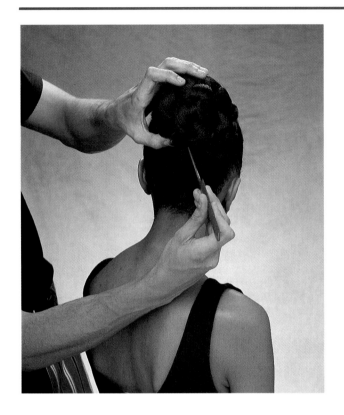

9 Secure the end of the braid at the same starting point in the back.

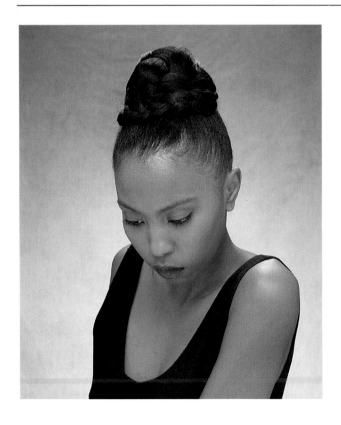

10 Once again check thoroughly for balance and to see that no pins are showing.

Note: Busy clients should be shown how to position and remove simple hairpieces like a chignon and/or braid.

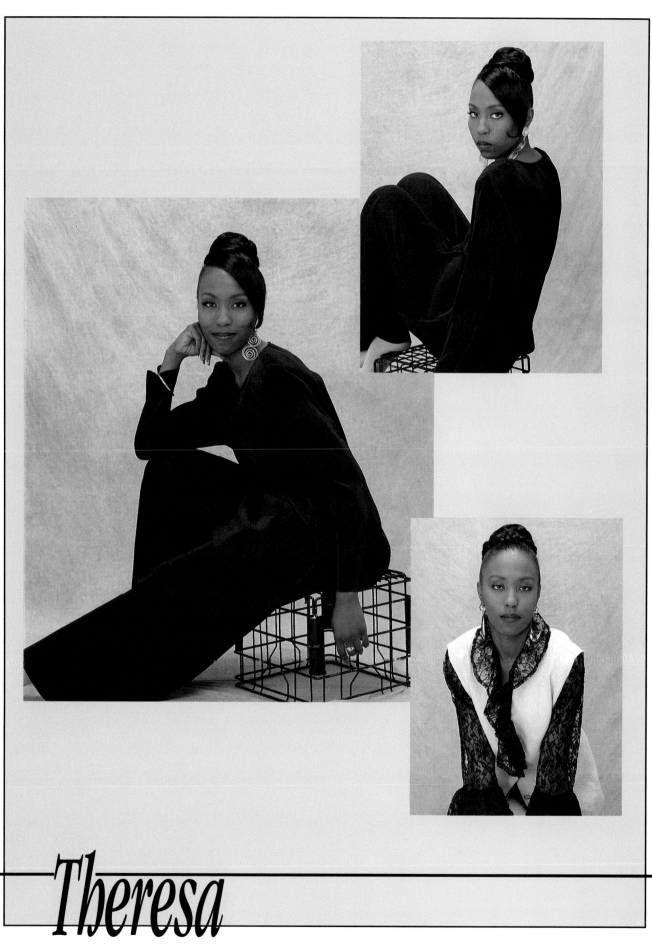

Theresa

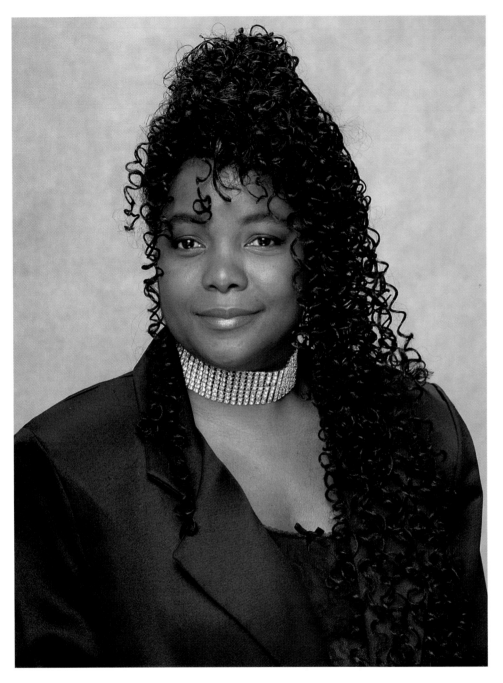

Long, luxurious curls can be easily attained by fashionable women who simply cannot grow their own locks. Faux extension by weaving is the answer.

No. *12* *Betty*

SERVICES

HAIR EXTENSION (WEAVING TECHNIQUE)

TECHNICAL REFERENCE NUMBER 110

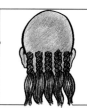

Most Black women have difficulty growing hair to long lengths. Harsh chemicals and products used to control excessively curly hair frequently cause the hair to break and hair ends to fray. Damaged ends must be trimmed often, preventing any hope of growing natural hair to extremely long lengths.

The client interested in added length usually opts for a hair extension attached by one of several effective methods.

The first and possibly the most important step when a client asks for a hair extension service is the initial consultation. There are several factors to be considered before the actual service:

a. How much added length does she want?
b. Should the extension be real or synthetic hair?
c. What color closely matches her own?
d. Should the added hair be curly, wavy, or straight?
e. How many extension wefts should be used for the amount of volume most adaptable to the client?

Betty's hair analysis is permanently recorded.

BETTY

HAIR ANALYSIS

Natural Texture: Wave ☐ Curl ☐ Kink ☑

Previous Chemical Service: Relaxed ☑ Straightened ☐ Colored ☐

Code:	1	2	3	4	5	6	7	8	9	10	
Porosity					✓						
Elasticity					✓						
Density					✓						
Coarseness					✓						
Hair Condition			✓								
Scalp Condition	✓										
Existing Gray	○										
Technical Reference Number	**110**										

Code based on a scale number 1–10

#1 = Good/Average

#10 = Poor/Abnormal

SERVICE RECOMMENDED

Shampoo and condition the client's hair so it is pliable, free from all residue, and easily handled.

PROCEDURE

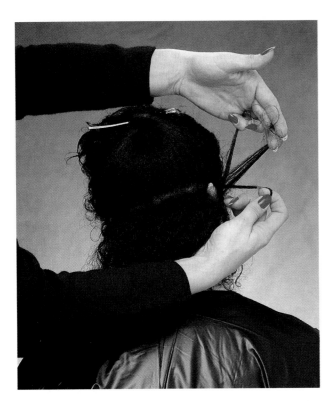

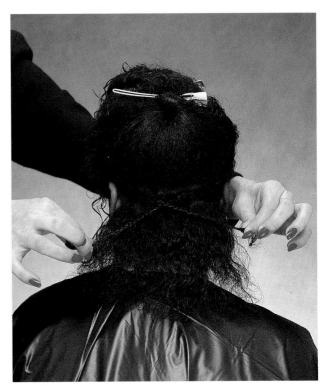

1 Part the hair from ear to ear just below the occipital bone. Make a very narrow three-strand French braid from each ear to center back.

2 Connect and secure the two braids at center back.

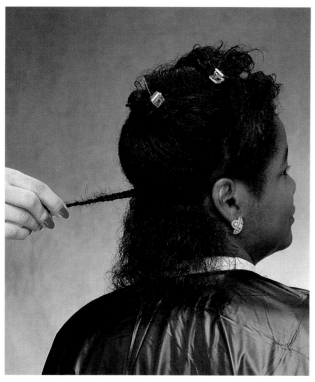

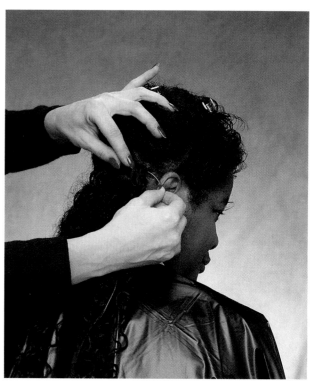

3 Braid the remaining ends to form one strand and to allow it to drop, becoming part of the back volume.

4 Start approximately one inch in back of the natural hairline and, using a curved weaving needle and thread at least two shades lighter than the natural hair, stitch the edge of the weft to the narrow braid.

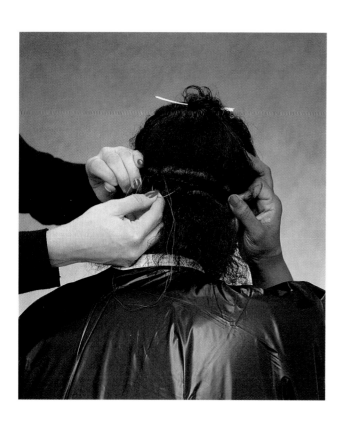

5 Work all the way across the head, attaching the weft from ear to ear.

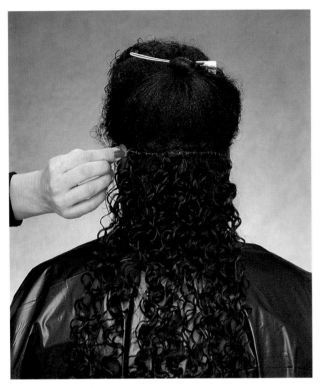

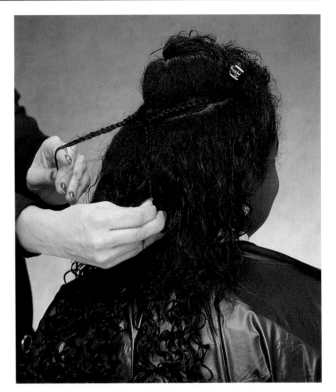

6 Secure the ends well and cut the thread leaving about a two-inch safety lead to prevent unraveling. The thread of a different color can easily be seen for easy removal when necessary.

7 Make two more partings approximately three inches apart, working from nape to the crown. Make narrow braids as in the first ear to ear parting and use the same attachment technique.

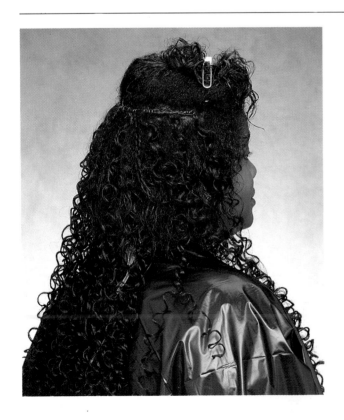

8 Usually two or three partings in the back give sufficient volume for a luxurious hairstyle. If the natural hair is sufficiently voluminous in the top and front no hair wefts should be added.

Note: Your clients should be made aware, if they do not know, that hair extensions are easily cared for with some simple instructions for shampooing. They are also easily removed or resecured as the natural hair grows.

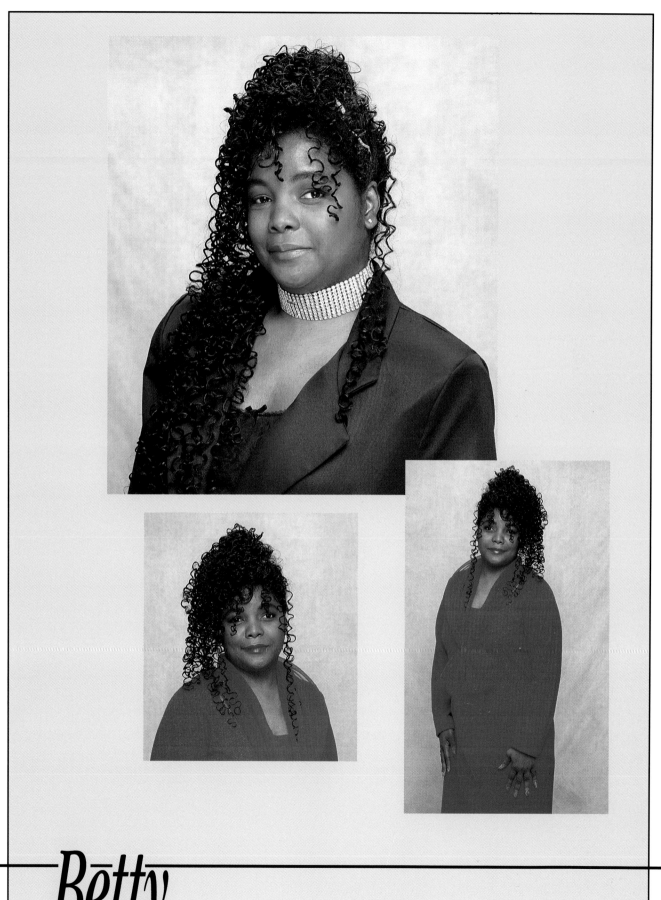

Betty

Glossary

HAIR COLORING TERMS

A

abnormal	condition of being less than normal, irregular
absorb	take in and hold fluid
abundance	plentiful, ample
abuse	misuse, improper use or application
accomplish	to complete, finish entirely, execute
adaptable	ability to change, conform easily
advent	a coming, approach
African	a native to Africa
African-American	person born in America of African ancestry
air-formed	style formed using blow-dryer and comb
air-styling	formed by hand-held blow-dryer and comb
airy	light and lacey
ammonia	compound containing nitrogen and hydrogen, soluble in water
ammonium thioglycolate	ammonia added to thioglycolic acid to form a compound
ample	sufficient in size or scope
analysis	examination of hair to determine condition and quality
appliance	electrical tool used in hairstyling
applicator	a brush, stick, swab, or container used to apply a substance
artificiality	not genuine, not from nature
artistic	skilled in various arts or crafts
assuming	to take for granted
attaining	to achieve, accomplish
average	general estimate based on comparison

B

balsam	a substance obtained from trees and plants used in hair conditioners
bangs	hair arranged on forehead
barrel	round cylinder
beneficial	to make good, advantageous
block	precisely dividing of hair for perming
blow-dryer	hand-held instrument for drying hair
blunt	straight cut without elevation
bob	short, blunt haircut
bonding	to fuse together
braiding	to weave or intertwine hair
breakage	broken or damaged hair
brittle	damaged and fragile
burning	skin affected by excess heat

C

camouflage	to disguise
Caucasian	relating to the white race of humankind as classified by physical features
casual	without formal design
challenge	obstacles/goals
choice	preference
characteristics	peculiar qualities of a person or thing
cholesterol	a solid found in all animal fats
chemical	inorganic elements other than those of carbon
circular	round
coarse	loose or rough in texture
compatible	existing together in harmony
color deposit	a color pigment that enters the hair cortex
corn rowing	term used for narrow braids on the scalp
cosmetic	beautifying; improving beauty, particularly that of the face and skin
coating	covering of the surface without penetrating

cortex	middle layer of hair made up of cortical fibers
confident	self-reliant, ability to feel in control
coil	to form rings or spirals
collagen	fatty substance
color level	hair color stages from one to ten
color lift	make natural hair color lighter
conceal	hide or disguise
concentrate	intense focus/deep thought
conform	to make of the same form or character
consumer	one who uses services or commodities
contemporary	currently existing or occurring
consultation	discussion of two or more persons with a view of some decision
corona	technical term for various things bearing some resemblance to a crown
curling iron	heated implement for styling hair
curl re-formation	changing the structure of the natural hair

D

damaged	impaired, injured
dampness	moist, humid
decolorize	removal of color
detectable	act of finding out what is concealed
deposit	application to the hair
density	number of hairs per square inch on scalp
demi-permanent	temporary, not lasting
design	shapes, lines creating an artistic unit
detergent	cleanser
detect	to uncover, expose
developer	activator
dictates	demands, influences
diminish	gradually become smaller
disorders	disturbs, interrupts

dissolving	liquefying
directional	course or line in which anything is directed
disulfid bonds	bonds found in cystine links of hair
disadvantage	that which prevents success or renders it difficult
discretionary	left to a person's own judgment
distribute	to divide into parts or portions
dreadlocks	twisted hairstyle worn by Rasta culture

E

effective	being solved in a satisfactory manner
elasticity	the ability to stretch and return to original form or length
electric	charged with electricity
elegance	refinement, grace, polish
eliminate	to set aside, omit
emphasize	stress a point or feature
end papers	used to protect and control hair ends when wrapping a p
enhance	intensify, make greater or more attractive
enzymes	protein substance produced by living cells
equalize	to adjust, make equal
essential	indispensable, a must
ethnic	relating to a people or race with common physical and cultural traits
excessively	beyond the usual or average
examine	to inspect, observe closely
exclusive	without admission of others, the only one
execute	to perform, complete
expertise	skilled knowledge or talent
extension	a lengthening or expansion
exotic	extraordinarily beautiful or different in nature

F

fabric	the principle structure of anything
face frame	hair that surrounds or frames the face
factors	parts or elements that make up the whole
fashionable	current, acceptable trend
faux	not natural; fake; manmade
finger styling	hair arranged without comb or brush, using fingers
finger waved	shaped or molded into waves while the hair is wet
fixative	a substance that sets, holds, or retains the hair in place
fibers	thread-like bodies of which animals or plants are composed
flaking	peeling or scaling off
flat	without elevation or depression, one dimension
flatter	to emphasize one's best features
foam	froth, aggregation of bubbles formed on surface of certain liquids by agitation
formation	creation, shape
formula	prescribed ingredients or components
formulated	created by use of a specific formula
fray	rub away, unravel
frazzled	a slang word for being exhausted
French braid	a three-strand braid executed near the scalp
fundamental	root, basis, foundation
fused	melted, dissolved

G

generic	of, or pertaining to, genus, distinct from the species or from other genus
genus	assemblage of species possessing certain characteristics in common
grease	a protein substance, animal fat

H

hair clips	metal or plastic clips used to hold pin curls or rollers in place
hairline	the exact place where the hair on the head meets the skin of the face or neck
hair picks	thin plastic cylinders (like toothpicks)
hard press	straightening the hair by using a hot iron on both sides of a strand or pressing the same strand two or more times in one operation
hot comb	a metal object for the purpose of straightening or relaxing curly hair; a cylindrical barrel in which metal teeth are set
heighten	to increase, intensify
heritage	that which is inherited, ancestral
high-lift	hair extending away from the head form
hone	to sharpen, to make sharper
hooded dryer	appliance for drying the hair having a hood that is placed over the client's wet hair from which heat and air are emitted
hot irons	a hand-held appliance, having barrels or tongs used to straighten or rearrange hair when heated
hot rollers	heat-resistant rollers preheated electrically and used for styling dry hair
hydrogen bonds	cross bonds in the hair that temporarily dissolve when wet

I

illustrate	to make clear, visual explanation
implements	tools or small appliances used in a trade
indentation	recess, depression
ingredient	component, compound, contents of a mixture
initial	first, the beginning
innovate	to uniquely create, change, or alter
insert	to set in, go within
introductory	in the beginning, to introduce or insert
interior	inside a perimeter, within a limited space
iron curling	curl the hair using heated, pronged curling irons

J

K

kinky	twisted, tightly curled, coiled
knowledgeable	educated, well informed

L

layering	cutting hair at various lengths throughout
lesions	irregularity on the skin or scalp; injury, an open sore
lifestyle	status, choice of environment, activity, the way one lives
limitation	restriction, boundary, within accepted bounds
lubricate	to soften with an emollient or oily substance
luster	shine, brightness, reflective quality
luxuriant	above average in comfort, quality, and appearance

M

maintenance	upkeep, perpetual care
manipulate	to handle, operate with hands on
Marcel iron	a small-barrel hot iron for making waves and/or curls in the hair, named for the inventor Marcel Grateau
mechanics	science of motion and force, physical structure or mechanism
medium press	a term given to the process of heat relaxing hair on only one side of a strand
mesh	to blend together
method	procedure, orderly manner of executing a project
minimal	small amount or degree
moderate	restrain from excess, limit
mode	manner, method
molding	to form, cast in a mold
moisture	wetness, dampness
molecules	small units of matter
mulch	blend thoroughly, mix together
mushy	damaged, oversoftened

N

natural	not artificial, produced by nature
neutralize	to destroy or render a substance inactive
no-base	a sodium hydroxide relaxer product that needs no prior protective application to the scalp
nonoxidizing	a tint or haircolor product that does not oxidize due to added developers such as peroxide or ammonia
nonperoxide	a haircolor product that deposits color without a proxide additive, has no lifting power
nucleic acids	organic compound important to living body cells

O

occipital	a bone at the base of the skull, often used as a position for parting the hair in preparation for cutting
omit	disregard, leave out, to not include
on-base	a roller or perm rod positioned in the center of a sectional space
opts	chooses, selects, prefers
oval	oblong, elliptical, egg-shaped
oversized	larger than usual, more than average in size

P

partial	not complete, a part of the whole
page boy	a long hanging hairstyle turned under at the perimeter
particular	careful, discriminating, specific
pattern	design
peroxide	H_2O_2, an oxide (oxygen) developer used in bleaches and tints
penetrate	to invade, to absorb, go into
perming	short term for permanent waving of the hair
permanent	when used in relation to hair care it means longer than temporary, will not shampoo out
pigment	the coloring matter found in human hair and skin
perimeter	outer edge
perm lotion	a liquid formulated (9.2 thioglycolic acid) for use in changing natural hair structure

perspiration	sweat, moisture excreted when the body is overheated
phenomena	out of the ordinary, often having no logical explanation
placement	positioning
powder bleach	a fast acting bleach product (high volume)
process	progressive course, the way in which something is done
preheat	heat prior to using
presoftened	weakened prior to a tint application
professional	as opposed to a novice, licensed to perform a skill
problem	a complication that hinders routine operation
protective lotion	a lotion used to protect the skin from chemicals contained in some hair care products
pressing	a term given to the use of heated implements for the purpose of relaxing curly hair
pressing oil	a light penetrating protein used to protect the hair from excessive heat during pressing or iron curling
predetermined	a decision made in advance
practicality	a conservative approach
pricy	a term used when services or products are unusually expensive
procedure	the orderly manner in which a project is executed
premature	before its allotted time
preferred	first choice
proficient	well qualified, competent
positioning	specific placement
primary	first step, basic
porosity	quality of being porous; capable of being penetrated
pliable	flexible, easy to handle
porous	loosely woven, having many openings in which moisture can enter
pH	potential hydrogen, the scale measuring degree of alkaline or acidity
profile	side view
protrusion	extending out of a solid form
prominence	center of attention, most noticed, featured
prudent	conservative judgment
protein	fat from animals

potential	possibility
pressing comb	a heated implement called a hot comb used for temporarily straightening excessively curly hair
preliminary	introductory or preparatory
practice	to do repeatedly
prior	before

Q

quality	distinguished, high rank, superior
quick service	fast, short-term methods and tools used to effect a hairstyle in a short amount of time

R

Rastafarian	a follower of a certain tribal African belief
receptive	open-minded
recession	a letdown, a time of economic recess
rectangular	quadrilateral figure having all right angles
reinforce	to strengthen
refinement	free from impurities
re-form	to force the hair into unnatural formation
relax	in hair-related terms it means to remove some or all of the existing natural curl
releasing	letting go, emitting
respond	react
reposition	to change from original position
resistant	not responsive
restore	put back to original condition
residue	a buildup of dirt and foreign matter
restructure	change the natural structure
retain	to keep
ringlets	tiny, full circle curls
rollers	tools for directing or styling wet hair
rotation	orderly change of position

S

saturate	wet completely
scorching	heating sufficiently to make a brown mark, near burning
scrape	abrade the surface
secure	hold tightly
semi-permanent	less than permanent, more than temporary
shrink	become smaller
sheen	a shine from a smooth surface
silking	making hair smooth
simulate	to copy
simplify	to make easy or uncomplicated
simultaneously	at the same time
skeptical	in doubt, without complete trust
skillful	exceptionally good at a craft
shiny	reflective
sleek	smooth
smoothed	surface made level
sodium hydroxide	a strong alkali formula used for straightening or relaxing curly hair
soft press	the practice of heat relaxing hair on only one side of each strand
solution	liquid mixture
span	to reach from one side to the other
sparingly	using a minimum amount
sparse	thin, not dense
special effects	special attention to detailing
specific	exact
specialized	highly developed skill in one service
specified	definite instruction
split ends	ends of the hair are frayed
spray	a fine liquid mist
squeeze	hold with pressure
stabilize	to make safe from undesirable change

stimulation	to make more active
straightening	a process to make excessively curly hair straight
stringy	separated as multiple strings
structure	foundation
static	electricity caused by friction
styling lotion	a substance used to assist in styling hair
stylish	in vogue, fashionable
subsection	a large section divided into smaller areas
sufficient	quite enough
surface	the outside, the top
synthetic	not from nature, made of manufactured material
system	a defined routine

T

tease	to push layers of hair from the ends towards the scalp
technical skill	a particular talent
techniques	ways of executing a project
technical	detailed, mechanical
temporary	for a limited time
tedious	time consuming
tendency	a leaning toward, an acquired habit, a natural trait
tension	held firmly, stretch
tensile	strength
texture	feel and look of fabric (hair)
thermal	heat
thermal styling	styling hair with heated implements
texturize	related to changing the natural structure of the hair either by cutting or curling
therapeutic	relaxing, healthy
triangular	a space having three connecting sides
transfer	move from one position to another
towel dry	to remove excess water from the hair by using an absorbent towel

treatment	as related to hair, a beneficial conditioner
trim	to remove excess length
transparent	an application that can be seen through
typical	average, usual

U

uniform	evenly formed
unique	one of a kind, different

V

various	many
vent brush	a bristle brush having a vented base
vertically	straight up and down, as opposed to horizontal
vitamins	nutrition supplements
virgin tint	the first time natural hair is chemically colored

W

weaving	a term given to adding length to natural hair by stitching wefts at regular intervals
wefts	hair, either synthetic or human, sewn in strips ready for attachment
wet look	a styling product that makes the hair appear to stay wet
withstand	tolerate
wrap	roll, wind

X
Y
Z

zigzag	an angular, uneven parting in the hair

Part III

FINISHED STYLES

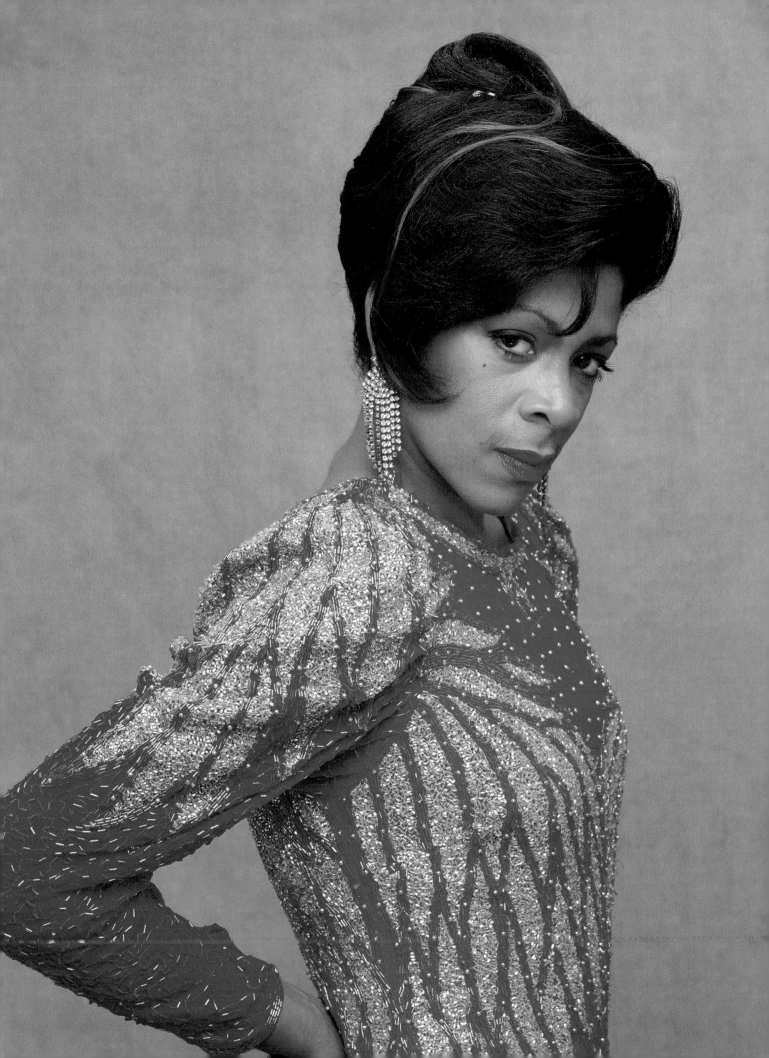

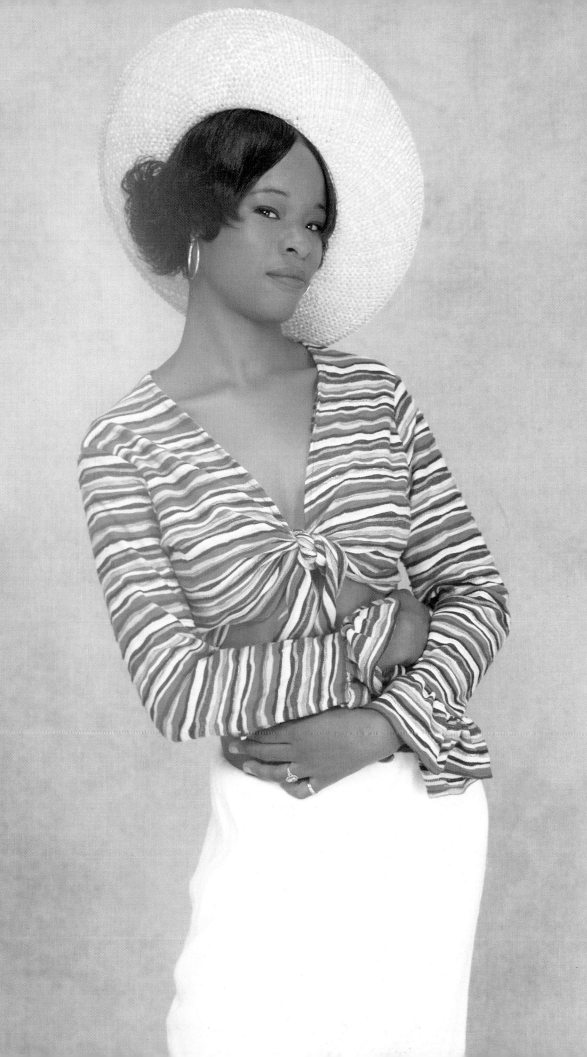

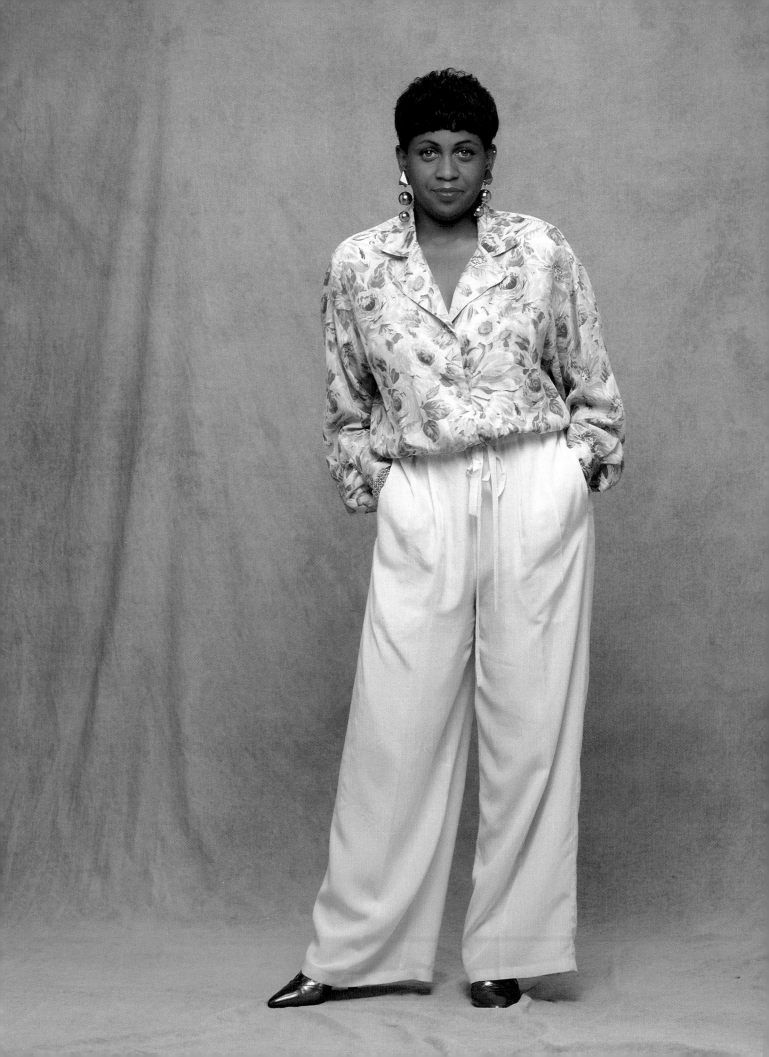

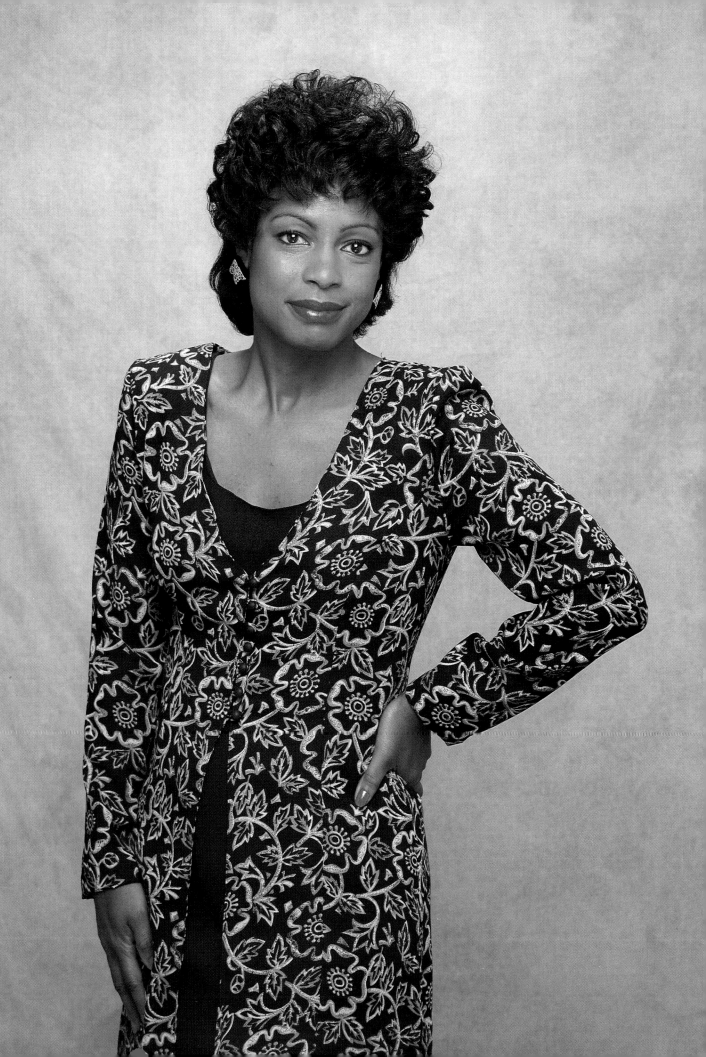

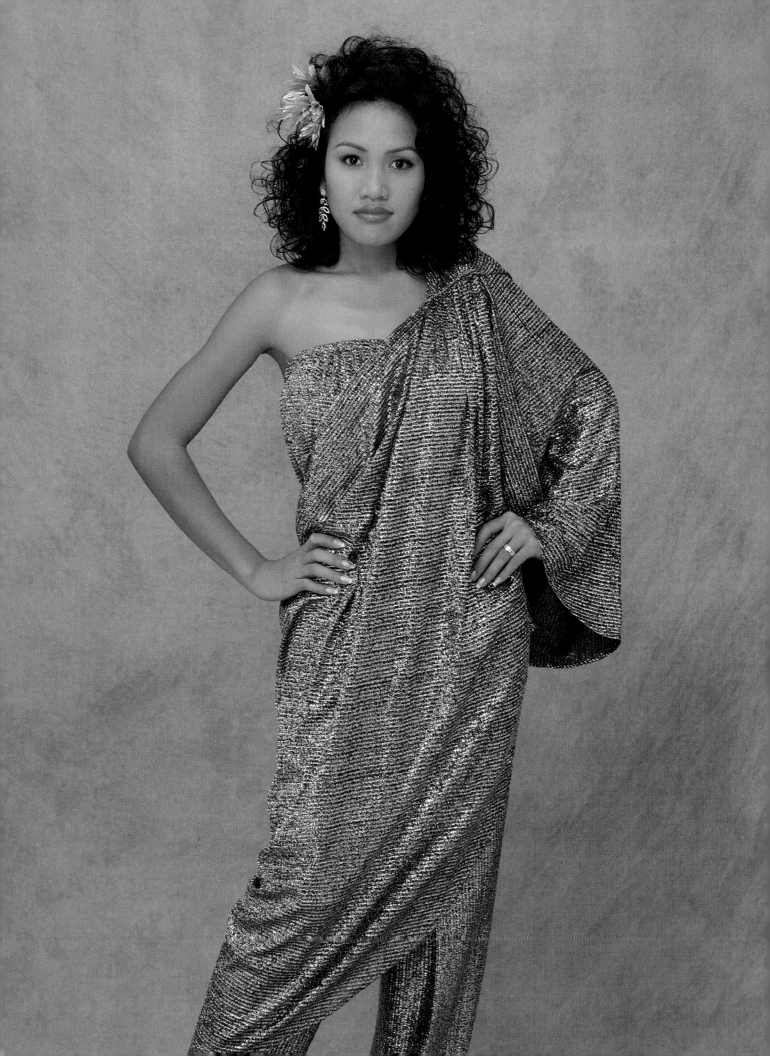

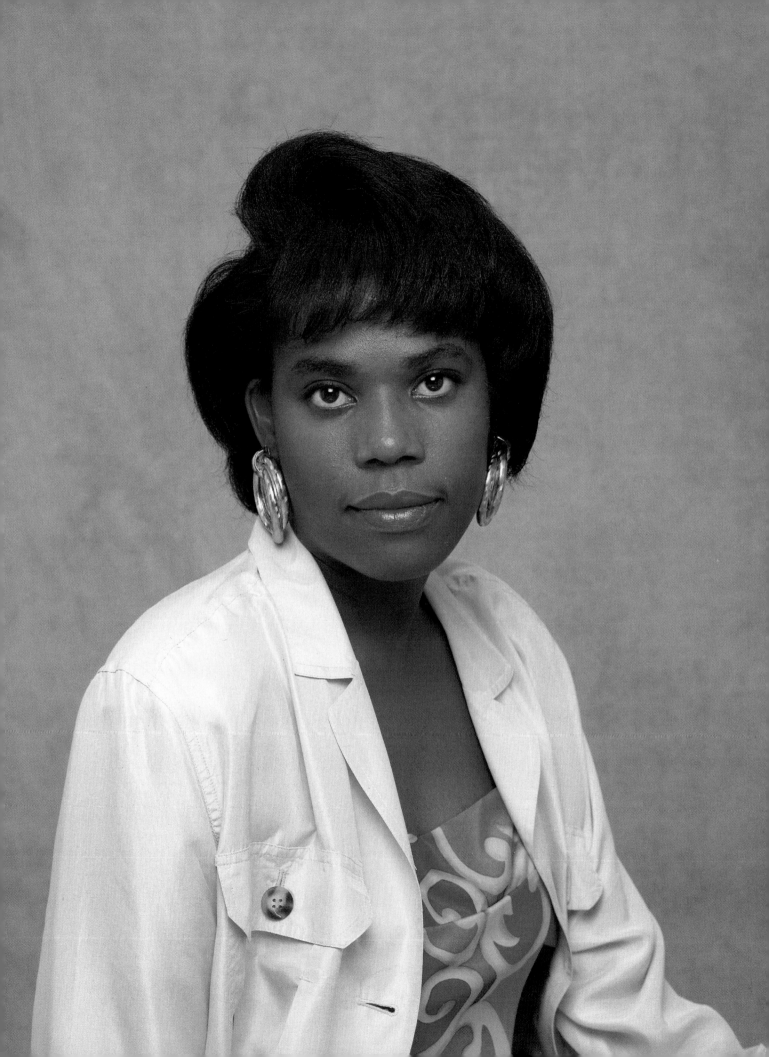

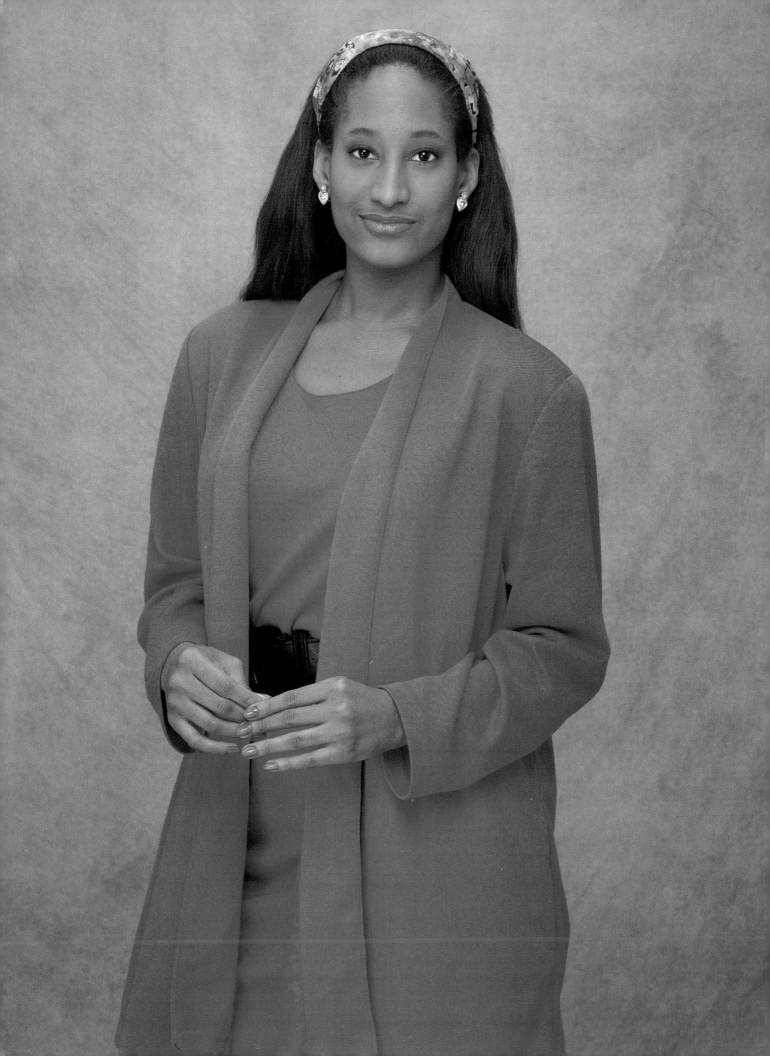

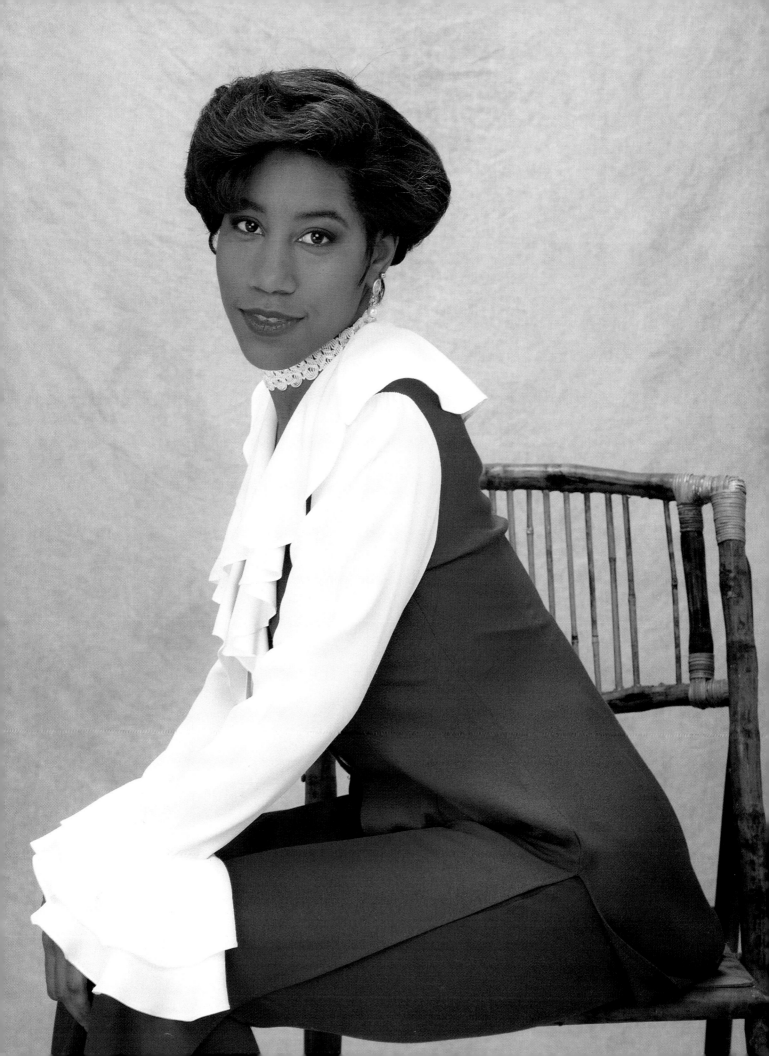

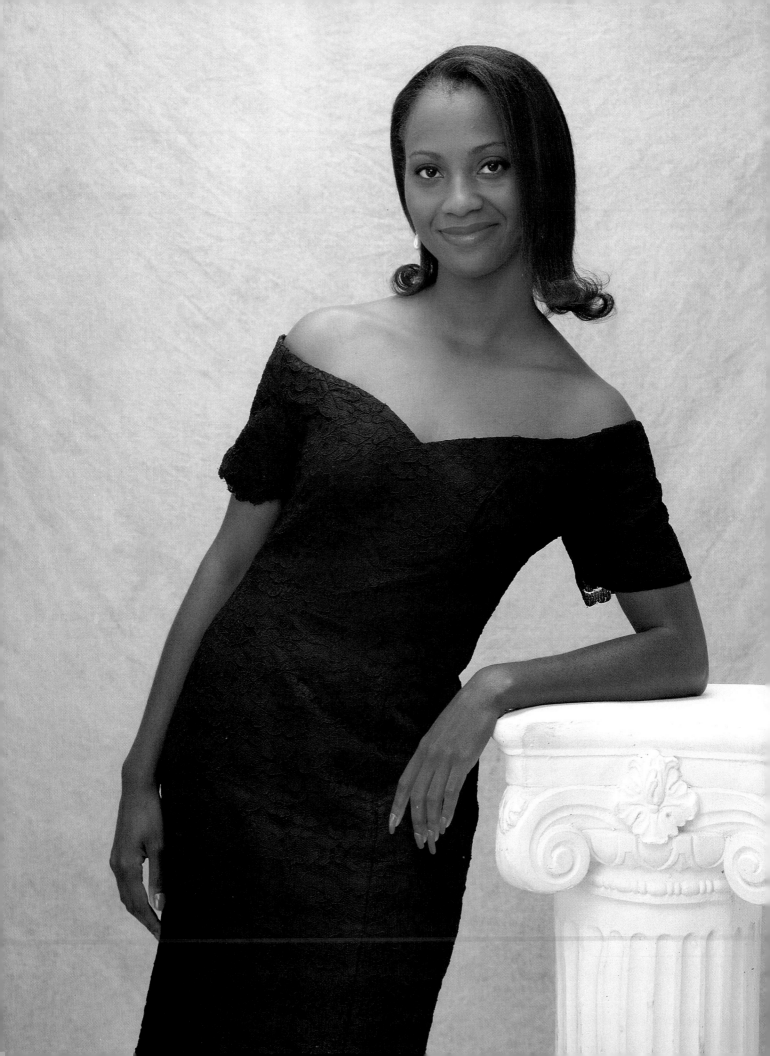

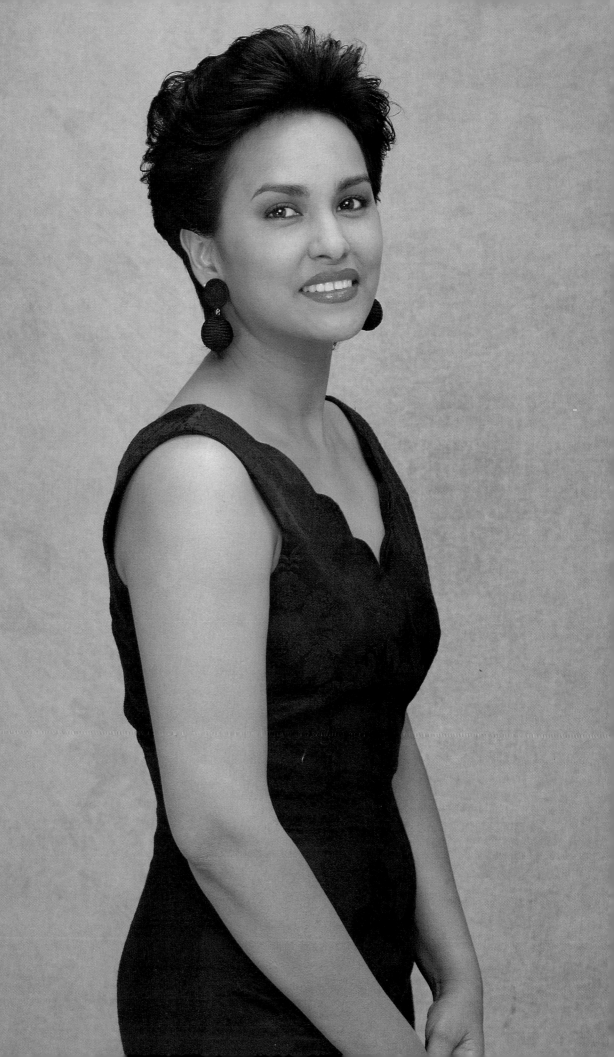

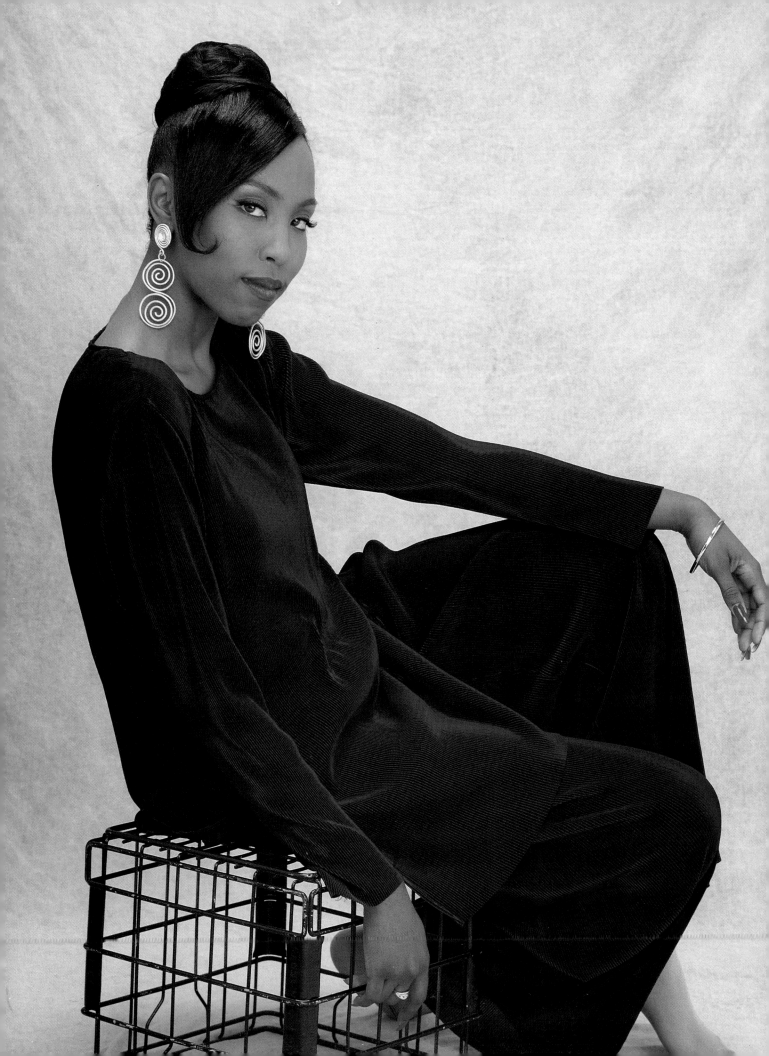

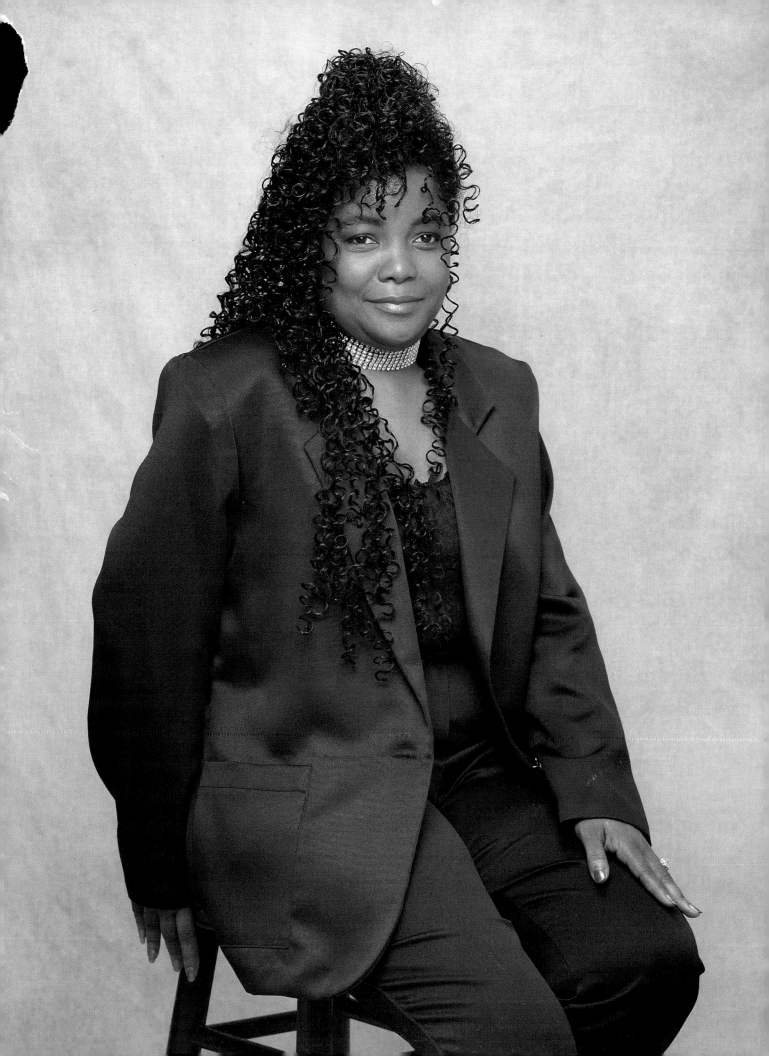